MY
BELLY

MY BELLY

Translated by **LUCY MOFFATT**

Hilde Østby

Exploring Why It's So Hard for Women to Love Their Bodies

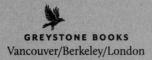

GREYSTONE BOOKS
Vancouver/Berkeley/London

First published in English by Greystone Books in 2024
Originally published in Norwegian by Kagge Forlag as *Mageboka:*
Sju steg mot å like kroppen din, copyright © 2021 by Hilde Østby
English translation copyright © 2024 by Lucy Moffatt

24 25 26 27 28   5 4 3 2 1

Greystone Books Ltd.
greystonebooks.com

Cataloguing data available from Library and Archives Canada
ISBN 978-1-77840-000-1 (pbk.)
ISBN 978-1-77840-001-8 (epub)

Editing for English edition by Jennifer Croll
Proofreading by Alison Strobel
Cover and text design by Belle Wuthrich
Cover illustration by sini4ka / Shutterstock

Permission for the poem by Kristin Storrusten on page 68
granted by the author. On page 132, the poem "Love After Love" from
The Poetry of Derek Walcott 1948–2013 by Derek Walcott, selected by
Glyn Maxwell. Copyright © 2014 by Derek Walcott. Reprinted by permission of
Farrar, Straus and Giroux in the U.S., Macmillan Publishers in Canada, and Faber
and Faber Ltd in the UK and Commonwealth. All Rights Reserved.

Printed and bound in Canada on FSC® certified paper at Friesens.
The FSC® label means that materials used for the product
have been responsibly sourced.

Greystone Books thanks the Canada Council for the Arts, the British
Columbia Arts Council, the Province of British Columbia through
the Book Publishing Tax Credit, and the Government of Canada
for supporting our publishing activities.

This translation has been published with the financial support of NORLA.

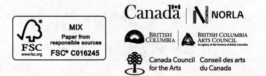

Greystone Books gratefully acknowledges the xʷməθkʷəy̓əm (Musqueam),
Sḵwx̱wú7mesh (Squamish), and səlilwətaɬ (Tsleil-Waututh) peoples on
whose land our Vancouver head office is located.

The good person
Walked past me on the street
And she looked perfectly ordinary
ANNE HELENE GUDDAL

Contents

Identify the Problem

A STRANGE ANNIVERSARY, WHEN I REALIZE SOMETHING HAS BEEN GOING ON BEHIND (OR RATHER IN FRONT OF) MY BACK

I'VE ALWAYS HATED having my picture taken. And this was a particularly important photograph. UK broadsheet the *Times* wanted an author photo of me and my sister for an interview. I'd spent the two-hour flight from Oslo to Berlin dreading it and had landed just a few hours before the scheduled shoot. The photographer was already setting up her equipment in a corner of the hotel lobby, fixing two lamps on stands and leaning some white screens up against the wall. Everything was in place to ensure that the lighting would be perfect. I said hi to my sister Ylva, who'd arrived at the hotel earlier, and went in to see the stylist, who was waiting for me in another room with a suitcase full of cosmetics. I barely had time to get changed and fix my hair before it was time to go down for the shoot. That day we were launching the German edition of our book about memory, *Adventures in Memory: The Science and Secrets of Remembering and Forgetting*; and on top of that, the *Times* wanted to write a double-page spread about the English edition. So they'd sent a photographer to our hotel in Germany. Only a fool would turn down that kind of publicity! But then there was the photo... If I'd known that this picture would push me into going for a winter dip in Oslo Fjord; selling half my clothes; doing hip-hop dance with a bunch of middle-class housewives; and learning about hormones and stress responses, happiness, and the origins of the human body, hermit beetles, and supernovas—if I'd known that I would turn my entire life upside down because of something that happened in a sterile German hotel on a perfectly ordinary Tuesday in November 2018, perhaps I'd have felt a bit more positive about it.

We sat beneath the harsh lights for more than an hour as the camera quietly clicked away. We smiled in a way we hoped looked intelligent, turned our faces a fraction of an inch to the side, raised our chins and lowered our chins whenever we were told to. And the whole time, I could think of only one thing: what does my belly look like? *That* is what was on my mind when I was having my photograph taken for the *Times*, for an article about a book we two sisters had written together, a book on a topic that had nothing whatsoever to do with my belly, or any aspect of my appearance at all, actually. I breathed deep, pulled in my stomach, tugged my clothes out, tried to smile. Luckily, I'd bought a huge sack of a dress on my way to the hotel. I felt confident that I'd probably manage to hide my body, sitting there in my tent. As I posed stiffly for yet another shot, I thought with some envy of male authors. Did this kind of thing occupy their thoughts *when* and *if* they simultaneously launched an English and German edition of their book? I couldn't quite picture Jon Fosse in the same situation: "Is my shirt too tight? Is my belly sticking out? Has my makeup started to run—no, luckily—my hair...how's my hair ...oh no, I forgot my belly, I breathed!" But what do I know?

The article didn't come out for ages, but when at last I held the newspaper in my trembling hands, I was able to confirm the only thing that mattered: you couldn't see my belly.

IT WASN'T UNTIL two years later, when I was about to turn forty-five, that I realized I was approaching an anniversary. I'd had a constant in my life for almost as long as I'd lived, and that was what the picture in the *Times* had made clear to me. Just before my birthday I sat holding the yellowing newspaper in my hands and knew that this anniversary had to be commemorated— but how? How *do* you celebrate the fact that you've hated your own belly for exactly thirty years? Which means, by the way, that I've hated my belly for the lifetime of an adult human being! If my belly hate was a person, she'd be old enough to have completed a lengthy education *and* given me grandchildren.

I did some calculations and found out that if I'd channeled all the energy I've wasted on hating my belly into writing books (a pretty sensible use of my energy, if you ask me), I would undoubtedly have managed to write a truly major work, on the scale of Marcel Proust's *Remembrance of Things Past* or Karl Ove Knausgård's *My Struggle, Vols. 1–6*. Without wishing to make too many assumptions about the inner lives of others, I don't believe either of those gentlemen can possibly have spent as much time hating their bellies as I have. If they had, they wouldn't have had enough time or energy left over to write seven thousand vividly told pages about small-town life in France at the beginning of the twentieth century and in Norway at the end of the twentieth century. And if they had hated their bellies as much as I hate mine, it's possible that every page would simply have been filled with: "I hate my belly, I hate my belly, why can't it just go away, will it help if I massage it flat? Or how about I just eat loads less than before, or better still spend the whole time starving—then it's sure to go away, oh god I'm two pounds heavier than this time last year, WHY can't I stay off the ice cream during summer vacation? My belly's sticking straight out—it's so repulsive!" And I doubt anyone would pay to read that.

THE STRANGEST THING about my belly hate is the *intensity* of my loathing. Another thing that surprises me is the way this hatred has become an absolutely integral part of me. And let me clear one thing up straightaway: When I use the word "hate," I really do mean hate—a word I reserve exclusively for Adolf Hitler and my belly.

The way my internalized belly hate works means that my belly is always the first thing I see when I stand in front of a mirror. The most important thing for me when I buy an item of clothing is how my belly looks in it. I've almost stopped noticing that I always adjust my clothes nervously and pull my belly in before I walk into a party or up on stage to give a talk. Only when I was about to celebrate my forty-fifth birthday did I realize that this shame about my belly, and this hatred, had become such an inevitable part of my life that I almost assumed it was something everyone must know about me; they must be able to tell just by looking at me, or be able to see it in that photo of me in the *Times*. Since it was the first thought on my mind whenever I entered a room, surely everyone must know I was a belly-hater, mustn't they? My belly hate is like a little dog that trots around after me wherever I go. Meeting new people at a party means having to introduce them to my belly-hate dog and me; going to job interviews means letting the little creature take a trot around my chair before I pick its leash up off the back of the chair and nervously leave the place. My belly hate can go quiet when I'm watching a film or a play because the auditorium is dark and people are always looking at something other than each other; but at a reception, a museum, a birthday party, even a funeral, my belly hate is back, standing beside me, sitting in my lap, wagging its tail if I've had a bad day, taking a nap when I feel good about myself. I've never entered a room without thinking about my belly. Maybe I should give it a name. Maybe I should call it Fido because this hatred has followed me so faithfully for the better part of my life.

THE IRONIC THING about this hatred of a random body part is that I've never wanted to earn a living from my own appearance. I've never once aimed to become a model, an influencer, an actress, or a fashion icon. Nothing in my dreams about life has ever indicated that I should be obsessed with my belly. Let me tell you a bit about myself: I was reading Roman comedies in Latin by the age of eleven, and if I had a crush on a boy, I'd mail him Shakespearean sonnets (it goes without saying that my advances were never successful). I was the kind of teenager who read Milan Kundera and Karen Blixen and Jorge Luis Borges, who got shivers down her spine listening to Shostakovich, and *had an opinion* about the twelve-tone composer Arnold Schönberg. Yep, I was a thoroughly precocious and all-round uncool teenager who went about dressed in her grandad's gray woolen pants, a baggy flannel shirt, hat, overcoat, and hiking boots. I wore zero makeup and had a nose ring. I was utterly scornful of all attempts at being sexy and pretty. And since this all was going on at the same time I was starting to read literature in earnest and had decided to become a writer, the people I should really have wanted to be like were my literary idols: So why didn't I long for a bushy mustache like Gabriel García Márquez, for the nose of Virginia Woolf, or fantasize about those enormous jug ears of Franz Kafka's? Why didn't I want to be like the people I genuinely looked up to? Why did I so specifically hate my belly?

Could it be, as many feminists think, that we are influenced by women's magazines and the prevailing body culture? Given my fairly sheltered life, steeped in culture and literature, that strikes me as almost impossible. Is it conceivable that I could have been influenced by the intellectually impoverished, toothpick-thin ideals of popular culture in my youth despite my protective blubber of sophisticated high culture? If so, how on earth did it happen? Can role models you don't give a damn about still have power over you?

I WAS A TEENAGER in the 1980s and I probably knew intuitively that, if you were aiming for stardom, you could forget about having a beer gut or even the tiniest roll of fat for that matter. I remember the actress Jane Fonda, one of the biggest idols of the day, who didn't just have a pancake-flat belly, but emphasized it by wearing an ultra-high-cut leotard, skintight and revealing. Not a single thick dark pubic hair or the tiniest camel toe in sight. It was almost as if Barbie and Barbarella and Jane Fonda were one and the same person: slick and smooth and perfectly formed, with flawless plastic skin and fluttering eyelashes. I noted how Madonna writhed for the cameras, how Claudia Schiffer's and Julia Roberts' pants hung from their hip bones, and although I didn't belong in their world, nor even wished to, they were still—astonishingly enough—role models of sorts.

But it's hardly surprising really: we're spongelike in our capacity to adapt to human society because we can't get by without it. In isolation, we humans are highly vulnerable, and our brain is a social organ. By the age of five or six, we are already internalizing standards and rules that we have picked up from the social situations we see around us all the time, to ensure that we can blend into the crowd we form part of. Before the age of six, we'll draw a picture and happily proclaim its brilliance, but after that tipping point in our development, we start to judge our drawings according to internalized standards.

We have absorbed what is right and proper from the world around us and have started to apply these rules to ourselves. And this isn't limited to drawings. We are hypersensitive to how other people behave, and the social rules that apply, as they show us both directly and indirectly. We humans live in constantly shifting cultures. And children, growing up in these finely tuned societies, grasp what is expected of them surprisingly quickly. This capacity for socialization, which we might call the "inner critic," serves as a social compass. The inner critic is what enables you to understand the rules that apply at a wedding (laugh and dance) and what you absolutely cannot do at a funeral (laugh and dance). It's what stops you from getting up and leaving a meeting where a colleague has wasted ten minutes you didn't have to spare telling everyone about his latest hunting trip and showing them photos of dead roe deer. Of course it makes sense to have an inner critic because it helps you to quickly learn the rules at a new school or workplace so you can blend in with everyone else. Your inner critic helps you to read situations and make jokes or look professional in a job interview.

The inner critic is here right now as I write this, and it's pretty ruthless: As I write, I'm generally thinking "Sorry for taking up your time" because my inner critic thinks I shouldn't write, that I should be silent, invisible instead. As you can imagine, that's a blessing and a curse, and of course the best thing to do is negotiate with it. That way, it can't throttle me, but at the same time I won't be so unleashed that I'll start behaving bizarrely.

A few years ago, I got a concussion and one of the oddest results was that I briefly lost my inner critic. I couldn't tell a joke to save my life but, more importantly, my behavior was completely uninhibited: I was no longer in harmony with my surroundings, I became slightly rude and odd, and behaved a bit childishly. A temporary injury of the temporal lobe like the one I suffered can rob you of a certain kind of social intelligence, making you less finely attuned to social norms. The thing is, we need to be switched on all the time if we are to understand the whole complicated game and all the unwritten rules we humans live by. The temporal lobe, which is located behind the temples, forms part of a network in the brain known as the executive function. This system is what gives us focus and direction in our daily lives; it's the place where we retrieve memories and associations, and assess the consequences of our actions; it's our working memory, which we use when we're thoroughly present in a situation—in fact, you're using it right now as you read this book. The temporal lobe blocks out inappropriate associations, noise, odd whims, and distractions, and it plays a role in humor. Understanding the social game is a big, complicated job that involves the frontal lobe, the large section of the brain right at the front of our forehead, which works in tandem with the temporal lobe in the executive function network.

YOU'RE PROBABLY THINKING I've gone off on a tangent here, but I haven't forgotten my belly; if I ever seem to have forgotten my belly, even for an instant, that's an illusion: I'm always thinking about it. Our inner critic is also switched on when we're thinking about what to wear in in the morning, because it makes sure that we won't look peculiar, with color combinations that are too jarring. My daughter, who's just about to start sharing her life with her inner critic—she's turned six—is still capable of leaving the house in a pirate costume and a pink sweater, with a peculiar braid in her hair, and rounding the whole thing off with a fanny pack and a pair of mismatched sneakers. This doesn't bother me much because in a few years' time she'll be obsessed with looking exactly like everyone else in her class. Take a walk past a middle school and you'll see what I mean. All those embarrassed kids in identical clothing offer a striking illustration of an inner critic in overdrive.

The point at which the inner critic makes its appearance and starts to tighten its grip is also the time when we become acutely aware of our own bodies and those of other people, an awareness that reaches a painful peak roughly in our mid-teens.

The hierarchies we live in are extremely important to us from an evolutionary point of view, because our ranking in the human community can be decisive out in the dangerous natural world. Social psychology studies have shown that we mostly compare ourselves to people we resemble. I'm more likely to compare myself with Julia Roberts than an Indigenous woman in South Africa, and although middle-class women in Oslo live a life more like my own, Jennifer Aniston is the one I look to—she's "perfectly ordinary" after all (apart from the fact that she can afford to spend hundreds of thousands of dollars on her body and appearance). She may even be more accessible to me than any of the women who live in my Oslo neighborhood. Although many of us no longer go to church in our culture, we still have altars: Our demigods speak to us in cinemas and on news websites; they live far away but shine out at us from our screens. It's perfectly natural, important, and—to some extent—vital for us to compare ourselves with others. So we do. We compare bodies. We compare bellies. We strive to imitate the demigods on the screen and fall short.

I WAS IN MY MID-TEENS, fifteen years old, when I found out that I, like Julia Roberts and Jennifer Aniston, was not supposed to have a belly. My belly should never stick out. Somehow or other, I'd picked up countless signals from the culture around me. Images and videos of people I didn't know or care about had started to dictate what I should feel about my own body. I ate as little as possible. I started doing sit-ups, a hundred a day at least. As I lay on the floor afterwards, hot and sweaty, I would run my fingers over my belly. My hip bones were supposed to stick up, sharp as the Rockies. Without even noticing it, I had decided what was normal, and this normality was starting to dictate my life. I compared myself to others, usually people I considered a bit better than me, people I should strive to emulate: flat-bellied Hollywood stars. I was obsessed with bellies, but so were teen magazines back then. Here's a quote from *Frida,* a Swedish magazine for teenage girls, in 1991— when I was sixteen years old: "Most of us probably dream of having a flat stomach." It went on to say that lemon water helps shrink bellies, and that you should spend the whole time thinking about your belly and constantly try to pull it in. Tips like these weren't unusual in the teen magazines of the 1980s and 1990s. Even today, I only have to go to my local supermarket to find the advice I need: "Here's how to get rid of dangerous belly fat" is such a frequent tabloid headline that it's hard to tell the different newspapers apart.

A study published in the *International Journal of Eating Disorders* revealed that more than 60 percent of respondents in a group of a thousand women aged between sixty and seventy were dissatisfied with their bodies and also classified themselves as slightly or very overweight. Eighty percent reported that they monitored their food consumption. When I first read this, I felt a profound weariness. Is the body hatred I cultivated as a fifteen-year-old seriously going to pursue me into old age? Will I sit there at seventy judging my own body to be failed and ugly? After wasting so much of my precious time up until now, am I also going to waste the precious years still left to me on hating my belly?

There is one woman in my life whom I've loved with a childish sense of unconditional happiness. My maternal grandmother. Whenever I visited my grandparents, who lived in a different town from us, I seized the chance to walk the few steps from the guest room, across the cold wooden planks of the corridor, and into their bedroom so I could clamber up into their double bed. The light fell in through the irregular 1940s window panes, which made it look as if the house lay on the edge of a glittering ocean. Once inside my grandparents' room, I crept happily beneath the morning warmth of my grandma's duvet and pressed myself close to her big, warm belly. During the day, I would lean against this belly as she sat knitting or darning socks. It was like a soft pillow. If I had to choose the most beautiful part of her, it had to be her belly. I don't believe this belly of hers was something she thought of as ugly or pretty; she had grown up on a farm and done physical labor during her youth. Nowadays she pottered around in her garden, kept house, cooked, and did handicrafts.

Her body had done its job; she was a working woman. But I can't know for sure what she thought about her belly, since she never spoke to me about her appearance.

Actually, no—there was one time, one single time she said something that involved values linked to body and appearance: I was thirteen and was wearing a brand new black maxi dress, sleeveless, with a broad black belt. I felt marvelous, almost grown-up. I had already started my period and I had a black dress; that's about as grown-up as you can get at the age of thirteen. I swished in and out of my grandma's house. It was summer, the morello cherries were ripening in the sun outside, and she was sitting on the sofa as usual. "Oh my, just look at that slender waist of yours," my grandma said, a touch of admiration in her voice, a kind of yearning that stayed with me. I knew at once that it was a good thing. And of course I didn't respond, "Oh my, look at that fat waist of yours" in a similarly admiring tone, because that's not an appropriate response. I'd already learned which standards applied.

MY DAUGHTER STANDS in the schoolyard, wild-eyed. She's a lion. It's Halloween. But almost all the other girls in her class have come to school dressed up as witches. "There's a cat!" I say encouragingly. "There's even a tiger! And a princess over there! Look, there are plenty of different costumes!" But most of the girls are witches and that's the only thing she can see now. She should have been a witch. When she came home from school recently with a wish list for Santa in her bag, there was only one thing on it. "I just want to be normel." So it's already started. She's scared of standing out.

People are much better at remembering negative experiences than positive ones, and when we compare ourselves with others who are a bit like us, the first things we notice are the areas where we feel we fall short. We overlook aspects where we are superior to the other person (all this, naturally, according to our own somewhat random scale). The reason for that is, of course, that it's much more important for us to remember the negative than notice the positive. Long ago, we humans would often find ourselves in much more dangerous situations than we do now, situations where our lives were at stake: back then, when our lives were much more closely entwined with nature than now, a trauma might involve seeing your best friend drown or get killed by a wild animal before you managed to find your own way to safety. It was crucially important to remember incidents like these so that you wouldn't end up in a similar situation yourself in future. All negative experiences lodge themselves more firmly in our memory than the positive ones to help ensure that we won't experience them again later in life. And the social hierarchies have been—and remain—extremely important to us. In fact scientists say hierarchies are so important that we have a special center in the temporal lobe dedicated to facial recognition for that very reason. Processing our relationships with other people and with ourselves is so vital to us that we expend a large share of our brain's precious energy on it.

One of the systems in the brain, the one that is activated when we are no longer focusing on anything outside ourselves, is known as daydreaming mode or the default mode network (DMN). This is where we anchor recollections in our memory and imagine what our future will be like. Strange whims and ideas can pop up when we are in this mode, and it is also here that our relationship with ourselves and others is processed. Considering what a calorie-guzzler the brain is—it requires vast amounts of energy—it is significant that we are apparently supposed to spend a full 50 percent of our waking hours daydreaming. Well, not daydreaming as in gazing lovestruck into the middle distance and thinking about our ideal wedding, but as in following associations and thoughts, running over that conversation with our best friend one more time, and planning vacations and dinners with our family. And we do all this in order to have a better life in the future, by learning from the negative in the past. Our memory is fallible because we don't need it to remember precisely what has happened, but rather to accumulate the building blocks we need in order to dream our way to a better future life for ourselves and those we love. Traumas and failures will take up more space than a happy or uneventful day because they are more important when it comes to planning how we do and don't want our life to be.

Neurologists classify part of this daydreaming as "brooding": This is when negative thoughts churn around like a washing machine on a slow cycle. All those thoughts about how ugly my belly is, for example—they run on a loop. This churning can cause depression. Yet it may also exist for a reason, to ensure that we don't repeat past mistakes. But how can a belly be a mistake? Perhaps my belly is simply the easiest thing to hate because it doesn't fit into our culture. Because somewhere between the fertility goddesses of the Neolithic age, with their gigantic boobs, enormous thighs, and sagging bellies, via the voluptuous, wobbly female flesh painted by Rubens and Rembrandt in the seventeenth century, and us today, something happened to the belly that left it at the very bottom of the hierarchy. Once upon a time, a little potbelly was a symbol of plenty and prosperity, of life itself, as illustrated by images of the Indian elephant god Ganesh, who sits there with his huge paunch, showering his worshipers with money. There are almost certainly cultures where bellies are still associated with beauty. But here in the West, they have come to symbolize poor self-control. Twenty thousand years ago in a totally different part of the world, I would probably have been proud of my own little potbelly, a symbol of abundance! I try to think of that when I undress at night, shameful and hunched over, sneaking past my husband to hide beneath the duvet as quickly as possible. Or when I pull on the skintight workout pants that leave nothing to the imagination, feeling as if I should apologize to my yoga class for exposing them to the sight of my belly. "Some time, some place," I try to say to myself, "this spare tire of yours would have been the most desirable thing anyone had ever seen." It doesn't help much.

In 1997, an extremely beautiful model appeared on the catwalks. Sophie Dahl was a so-called "plus-size" model—and the grandchild of author Roald Dahl too, by the way. She had enormous eyes, a charming doll-like face, and a zaftig body. She instantly became the darling of the fashion world, not so much because she set a new standard, but because she offered a kind of cool contrast to all the stick-thin models with their boyish hips and invisible boobs. Sophie was just as unattainable for me as Kate Moss (one of the stick-thin models) because she was strikingly beautiful and her weight was distributed in an exceptionally womanly fashion. Unlike me, she didn't have broad hips and an apple belly stacked atop two short, skinny legs. I'd have been happy if could've put on weight the way she did. If I could've had big hips and big boobs and still kept my own face, I'd have been happy to put on a bit of weight. But even my face changes when I pile on the pounds, becoming moonlike; and when I get over-weight I mostly end up with a big belly, not big boobs.

"Plus-size" models turn up more often these days, reminding us of the fertility goddesses of past eras. They make a single guest appearance then vanish again. It seems their mere existence is supposed to make us feel liberated, even though most of the women gracing magazine covers and film posters are still thin as a pin—indeed, no doubt about it, under-weight. But no matter who I look at—the exhausted mother of three airing her fat rolls on the beach, beauties like TV cook Nigella Lawson and Sophie Dahl (who has, by the way, slimmed down drastically since 1997), or body positivity activists posting big bodies on Instagram—I don't think any of this eases my own inner craving for a flatter belly. It's still there, even after exposure to hundreds of perfectly ordi-nary bodies, exhausted, stretch-marked, and wobbly. Plenty of body positivity activists are trying to spread precisely this message: They pose naked or in bikinis—paunches out—to serve as a counterweight. I'm pleased to see them in a way, but I'm not sure they do anything to alleviate my hatred of my own body.

DURING THE WHOLE of the summer I turn forty-five, I wander around the beaches of Oslo looking at other people's bodies. I mean, I'm there to swim, too, but at the same time I take the opportunity to look at other women. Most of them are perfectly ordinary in their own particular way: They're slim and *too* slim and pudgy and overweight, with belly fat and great bouncing breasts and rolls of fat beneath their bikini straps and cesarean scars above their bikini bottoms, stretchmarks on their thighs, and wounds and scars and injuries. That summer, I'd planned to wear a bikini. I bought a pretty rust-red one with gold details. If only my body was as pretty as the bikini, I'd be happy to strut about on the beach in it. But I just can't manage to think like one of the body positivity activists I follow on Twitter, who writes: "Put on your bikini. There: Now you have a bikini body!" I wear my emerald green one-piece instead and try to "see myself free" of my belly hate. If it's true that seeing skinny bodies makes me want to be thin, surely seeing lots of non-skinny, perfectly ordinary bodies must be enough to make me start liking a perfectly ordinary body, mustn't it?

Since I don't buy magazines or go to the movies more than a couple of times a year, and rarely if ever watch TV, I've probably seen far more normal bodies than model bodies. Yet those stick-thin bodies must still have set a standard for me that cannot be beaten out of me by looking at some unknown woman's extra roll or two of fat. At any rate, it doesn't work for me. That said, I'm extremely happy to see Lena Dunham on TV, simply because she's a clever, funny woman who's also good at talking about important, serious issues without being stick-thin. It certainly makes me happy to see different bodies and to see clever women in all shapes and sizes; I just don't want to be that different body *myself*. And of course it's great that Press—the youth wing of Norwegian Save the Children—awards an annual Golden Barbie prize to the advertising and media player that has made young people feel *worst* about themselves. The same organization has reported that 55 percent of children and young people want to change their appearance. Meanwhile, according to the Norwegian Media Authority's survey "Children and Media 2020," around half of thirteen-to-eighteen-year-olds have been exposed to social media ads promoting weight loss or muscle growth. We adults must tell them clearly that their role models may be the ones with the problem, not them.

A SURVEY OF ALMOST SIX THOUSAND university students in Gaza, Egypt, and Finland demonstrated something that had already been revealed by surveys in both Portugal and the United States. You might think that the most important factors for a positive image of one's own body would be exercise and healthy eating. But it is still possible to have a negative image of your body even if you work out and are thin by strictly objective standards (low body mass index); indeed, in some cases, negative body image intensifies as the person's BMI decreases. By and large, I've hated or been dissatisfied with my own body ever since I was in my mid-teens, even though my weight has fluctuated dramatically during that period. I have been extremely underweight and pretty overweight, but on the whole, the feeling has remained unchanged, and I have been at my very unhappiest when I have also been at my very thinnest.

The large-scale study of six thousand students revealed a perfectly clear trend: the factor common to people with a negative body image in different countries and regions of the world is *depression*. The authors write: "body image-depression links are supported by neurobiological investigations... brain areas involved in hedonic regulation may play a role for both body image and depression."

And just recently I found out what Jane Fonda was going through during that period when she was dancing and smiling her way through her workout videos. When I watched the HBO documentary *Jane Fonda in Five Acts*, it became clear that, as well as being a passionate political activist, she was also a person who had battled with bulimia all the way from puberty into her fifties.

"I was raised in the 1950s," she said. "I was taught by my father that how I looked was all that mattered. He was a good man, and I was mad for him, but he sent messages to me that fathers should not send: Unless you look perfect, you're not going to be loved."

Making workout videos that combined ballet and yoga financed her politically active husband's campaign and simultaneously gave her a route out of bulimia—a disorder triggered by the attitudes of her biggest role model, her father. Without making too many assumptions, I'm fairly certain her main objective was absolutely *not* to give a fifteen-year-old from Oslo the idea that the only important thing about women's bodies was a flat belly. Nonetheless, absurd as it may seem, her father, the famous actor Henry Fonda, did have a bit of a say over my body, here in Norway. Do I transmit that belly hate, inherited from Henry Fonda via Jane Fonda, to my own child? Not so long ago, my little girl strutted downstairs to the bathroom stark naked, shouting coyly: "Look, Mom, I'm yucky. I'm naked!" I drew a deep breath and said, as calmly as I could, trying to suppress the sinking sensation in my stomach: "You're the most beautiful girl in the world—naked, with clothes on, always." But how can I be sure that'll be enough? If Henry Fonda gave his daughter Jane the idea that she wasn't loveable if she wasn't beautiful, mightn't I be capable of doing the same thing? What kind of signals do I unwittingly send to my daughter? Does she see me standing there, tugging and adjusting my clothes in front of the mirror, pulling in my belly and holding my breath? Does she see that I'm looking at my own body, my own face, with a vague loathing? Does she hear my sigh of resignation as I pull one pair of pants off and put another pair on?

To drill right down to the heart of the problem: Did I once have a Henry Fonda in my life telling me how important my appearance was? Nope, my father was the opposite: When I was growing up, he gave me affirmation for what I thought and did, not how I looked. I have never once felt that he would only love me if I was a nice, sweet little girl. He discussed philosophy with me (he's a professor in the discipline), he played Shostakovich for me, he read Charles Dickens aloud to me at bedtime. I don't think he has ever even noticed what I wear. Not that I was a very elegant dresser, being a child of the seventies; I usually went around in second-hand corduroy pants and a home-made sweater. He has always said: "Don't be afraid to say what you think," and I never have been. I believe I have him to thank for the fact that I am an author and critic today. So why do I hate my belly? Why do I think this part of my appearance has any significance at all? Who made me think that way?

Some surveys conducted in Norwegian kindergartens reveal an unpleasant fact. Despite regulations requiring kindergartens to treat all children equally, irrespective of gender, that is not what happens. Both parents and kindergarten staff offer children affirmation based on some perfectly clear patterns. From the time they are tiny, girls are offered compliments and assurances about their appearance and their clothes, while boys are asked about what they've been doing. *Appearance* versus *action*. The trend is so clear that it can't be accidental. Although I have no way of finding out whether the same thing happened in my own kindergarten and my own school, I have to assume that it did: Long before I'd seen a single film or music video, long before I'd heard of Jane Fonda and Jennifer Aniston, long before social media and advertising billboards on street corners and TikTok stars—indeed, long before I'd read Franz Kafka and Milan Kundera—I had probably realized that what mattered for girls was their appearance.

I mentally rewind to that episode when my daughter strutted down the stairs, naked and coy, shouting: "I'm yucky. I'm naked!" I think about the way I answered her; I think about all the times I've whispered, shouted, murmured, "You're so beautiful ... don't you look lovely, honey ... that dress is so pretty." And I think about that time she clapped herself contentedly on the belly and said: "Just right! Look at that tummy, Mom. It's just the right size." When will she stop thinking that way?

I THINK I NEED TO CALL my belly hate something other than Fido. Perhaps it needs a name that signifies what a dark and dangerous dog it is; a dog that grows bigger and stronger the less food it gets—a dog that bites. A really ugly beast! Ragefeeder—that's what I'll call my belly hate. And now it's time to take it to the vet: it's time to put it down.

Know Your Enemy

I'M PREGNANT ONCE A MONTH

"ARE YOU PREGNANT?" the man before me blurted the question out, seemingly delighted on my behalf. Dressed in dark polo-neck and glasses, he was holding a glass of wine—we were at a party. I had a glass of wine in my own hand, was wearing a black dress, and until a few seconds ago I'd been feeling pretty good. Now it felt more as if I'd been drenched in a bucket of icy water, and all I wanted to do was stand stock still, frozen in the moment, so I could escape the inevitable aftermath. I found I had no ready answer, no joke or light-hearted quip that could draw the sting out of the situation, no standard response from the Handbook of Etiquette: "If a gentleman asks whether you are pregnant, the correct response is to punch him on the nose and, possibly, pour a glass of red wine over his head."

As I stood there in front of this much older man gulping back the tears (for although *he* was the one who had violated a dozen social codes, *I* was the one left feeling ashamed), I failed to say what I should have: "I'm just a bit fat right now and *really* premenstrual. As I'm sure you've heard, that's the worst hormonal hell known to humankind. Not only do the rise in progesterone and the drop in estrogen and serotonin in the run-up to your period make you puffy and gassy, but your body also retains water, making you swollen and bloated—and on top of *that*, the drop in serotonin increases your appetite for sweet things. Did I mention, by the way, that the increase in progesterone slows the digestive system, often causing constipation? Of course I look pregnant— I'm packing a poop the size of a seven-month fetus! How's your penis doing, by the way?"

I didn't say that. I just looked at him as if he'd shot me in the kneecaps, tears welling up and a hot flush of shame spreading across my face. I put down my wine glass and cast a last glance around the party, probably filled with the same emotion that Emperor Nero experienced back in 64 CE as he looked on in disbelief while Rome, the most fabulous city in antiquity, went up in flames in what is, to date, the biggest ever city fire in peacetime—apparently started by Nero himself. Unlike him, though, I wasn't remotely to blame for the fact that the party was crumbling to ashes before my eyes. I headed resolutely for the door and went straight home. Once there, I tore off the black dress, hurled it in the garbage without a second thought, grabbed a carton of ice cream from the freezer, and settled in front of the TV to watch a crap film.

IN THE YEARS SINCE THEN, I've been asked many, many times whether I am pregnant, almost always by men, generally men slightly older than me, generally in a congratulatory tone. Interestingly enough, no such concern was in evidence when I really needed it—when I was heavily pregnant for real and not a single passenger on the bus or streetcar gave up their seat for me. Maybe they were afraid I wasn't actually pregnant and didn't dare ask; maybe they'd heard about that guy who made a jerk of himself at a party twenty years ago and learned from his mistake. If so, what an irony.

THERE'S A REASON I REACT so forcefully to being asked whether my empty uterus is full: It's because something I'd assumed was discreetly tucked away and invisible, a part of my body whose primary purpose is to quietly get on with the business of digestion, looks unusual enough to provoke a comment. If strangers constantly pointed out that I had a weird nose or arm, it would be about as unpleasant as to be told the same about my belly. Most of us don't want to stand out too much, we want to look "ordinary" (so, in my case, like Jennifer Aniston). Being a wheelchair user and always getting comments and questions about why you have to use it must be infinitely more unpleasant than my belly experiences. Always feeling stared at because of the color of your skin must be equally disturbing. But the extra little sting in my case comes from the misplaced and awkward *joy*, the congratulations; this sparks a situation that could easily be reproduced in a film as a total clash in perceptions of the world, a true tragi-comic moment that wouldn't be out of place in a Woody Allen movie (if Woody Allen were the slightest bit interested in issues like this).

The social conventions linked to pregnancy and bellies have made me spend more time than I actually want to on thinking about my body and the fact that I'm a woman. But how do pregnant, premenstrual, and menstruating bodies really work? Perhaps I can make peace with my belly if I understand what's going on inside there, how it all works.

We don't all menstruate at the same time. If we did, the rivers would run red. But the fact that many people, mostly women of childbearing age, menstruate every twenty-eight days—exactly the same length of time it takes the Moon to orbit the Earth—created an historical association between femininity and the Moon, with its unpredictability and its apparently magical ability to control the tides.

Far back in time, the uterus fell victim to countless misunderstandings: Given its link to an activity as mythical and mighty as the creation of new life, it was blamed for the "disease" of hysteria (from the Greek word for uterus). Yes, from the days of the Ancient Greeks until well into the twentieth century, people commonly believed that the uterus (a large muscle capable of expanding to five hundred times its original size) could cause a state of psychotic irrationality. Obviously, there's a small grain of truth in this, since the menstrual cycle can trigger both minor depression and major aggression. Recent research on the menstrual cycle also shows that it can't just cause temporary irritability, anxiety, and depression, but can also alter the brain, leading to better spatial awareness early in the cycle than later on. In the same way, the capacity for creativity and problem-solving, memory, and empathy increases in the early weeks of the cycle compared with the last constipated days before menstruation. Luckily, I'm writing this difficult second chapter at the start of my cycle. Later on, everything descends into a chaos of depression and defecation.

Michelle Wolf's material on periods contains some of the funniest jokes I've ever seen told by a stand-up comedian: "You know that picture of Marilyn Monroe where her skirt's blowing up? Yeah, that wasn't an air grate, that was a period fart. Masturbate to that," she says, adding, "You also say things like, 'Why are you so emotional?' Well maybe it's the hormones or maybe it's the fact that I haven't shit in a week." I'd never heard anyone say any of this out loud before—I thought it wasn't allowed; I thought it was secret. So many aspects of our bodies can seem disgusting and shameful that the belly is just the tip of the iceberg. Our bodies and minds are constantly in motion; we produce and dispose of bloody tissue, retain water, and fine-tune our hormones—and do all this while simultaneously paying bills, conducting adult conversations, and following complicated recipes.

In other words, there's something fluid and unpredictable and treacherous about feminine bodies and inner lives, from our early teenage years right up until we reach the age of social death (menopause). If masculinity is a cliff, a solid structure, then femininity is like the sea, with a high and low tide.

I'm often expected to accept that I lack rationality just because I have a uterus and female hormones. But that's not true: *despite the fact that* my hormones mess with my spatial awareness and my mood, *despite the fact that* I'm like an ocean whose waves can suddenly tower ten feet in the air and drown random passersby, I achieved top grades in every single subject at school. The two things aren't mutually exclusive—and it's incredibly annoying for someone to claim that I'm irrational just when I'm in the middle of a premenstrual rage!

What I've realized is that the feminine body is subject to much greater fluctuations than the masculine body: it changes, becoming new and different all the time—it's actually a super-body! Comparing a feminine body with a masculine body does me no favors, making my advantages look like weaknesses. My body can transform itself from hard and thin to big and soft in record time. Much of my hatred of my body is linked to an intense need for control, a desire to keep my body steady, to transform it into a stable masculine body. And that, in turn, may be linked to my first experience of becoming a woman in puberty. That was when my body stopped being a boy's body. When I was ten, I could run just as fast as any other ten-year-old, regardless of gender. Ever since that first betrayal, I've never stopped longing to get back to that boy's body; I still haven't quite accepted that my body will not become like that again.

Instead, I'm subjected to a kind of guessing game, an advanced version of "Will the weather be good or bad?" Every day, I wonder what my body has in mind today, and how far it's planning to cooperate with me. All my detailed planning and careful organization of life in general can be challenged at any given time by my body's inability to obey orders. Why won't it do what I tell it to? Why doesn't it behave as if I was a man? Because I'm a *woman*! I find myself constantly surprised by the fact even though I've done one of the most extraordinary things a human can possibly do—give birth to another human being. That may be what makes the belly so scary and striking, perhaps especially for cis men: There's a place in my body where life is created! They observe my belly and see my superpower, see my might. All I see is a slightly protruding belly. It's tempting to think that all the misogyny in the world has a single source—this power that I possess but no cis man does. Sheer *uterus envy*, I guess.

THE ACTUAL PROCESSES of menstruation and pregnancy are among the most extraordinary things that can happen in a body. Roughly every twenty-eight days, the uterus builds itself up to receive a fertilized egg. But even if a fertilized egg does come floating down the fallopian tube now and then, it'll have a tough job forcing its way through the thickened uterine membrane. Ten to 25 percent of all fertilized eggs fail to attach, which is a way of guaranteeing that the successful candidates are capable of becoming viable babies. However, if the egg does manage to attach, the placenta will set about expanding the body's blood vessels to ensure ample access to blood.

The placenta is an entirely new organ and becomes a kind of hostage negotiator between baby and pregnant parent. It weighs about a pound by the time the baby is born, is expelled after birth and is then forgotten. But, as I say, it is an entirely separate organ that produces several as yet unidentified hormones, which protect both baby and parent. Research into why people develop cancer has focused on the placenta because we humans have to be able to cope with the placenta and fetus behaving like foreign bodies in *our* body. In order not to reject the fetus, the pregnant body must accept the "evil invader," and that is thought to make us humans more susceptible to developing cancer than many other species.

It isn't just the hormones that change the parent; after a pregnancy, small traces of the fetus can be found inside them. The fetus sends out stem cells, which can travel around in the pregnant body and reinforce existing tissue. They can even create new neurons in the brain, according to research from Arizona State University—and new brain cells are pretty rare (unlike cells in the rest of the body, cells in the brain are not renewed, with a few exceptions). Fetal cells can be traced in women aged ninety-plus—they apparently remain through the whole of their life, like a strange memento of the pregnancy. We don't know why the fetal cells travel around the pregnant body and settle in the organs, but it may be that the fetus sends out these stem cells to give the birthing parent the extra strength needed to cope with the postpartum period.

Pregnancy can be compared to an invasion, in that it develops in a similar way. Once the fetus has attached to the uterus, it sends out hormones that raise the blood pressure and blood sugar. This, in turn, increases the flow of blood through the uterus, ensuring that the fetus has access to sufficient nutrients. No wonder being pregnant is so exhausting! Put simply, during pregnancy, the body falls under the hormonal control of a foreign body armed with super placenta cells that invade it with fetal stem cells. Countless things can go wrong at any time during this process—not to mention the birth itself. Even in our modern era, eight hundred women still die in childbirth *every day.* This largely happens in countries where the health services aren't as good as in the industrialized nations—South Sudan tops the statistics, with more than a thousand dead mothers per hundred thousand births—but even in developed countries with good healthcare, women die in childbirth every year.

Humanity is close to the tipping point when it comes to the size of the child's head relative to the pelvis: We walk upright and that requires a narrow pelvis; at the same time, though, we're supposed to give birth to a child whose relative head size is the largest in the entire animal kingdom. And when the child comes out, its childhood is also the longest (relative to our lifespan) in the animal kingdom. You need only look at the cute little lambs that plop out in lambing season and almost immediately rise up on their thin, unsteady legs to grasp just how helpless we humans are in the very first hours—indeed years—of our lives; how dependent we are on each other.

I truly thought being pregnant was wonderful (although giving birth most definitely was *not*). I felt paleolithically powerful and wild. All this while the contents of my belly were being scrambled up and my organs were being moved around, and ended up getting squashed to make way for something incredible: a kind of parasite—a brand new human being! For the first time, my prominent belly was quite natural and I could beamingly answer yes every time anyone asked me if I was pregnant. Suddenly the world and I were on the same page about what my body was. My inner critic had a brilliant time, in other words, because it wasn't constantly having to adjust to the people around me. I bought myself a pale-blue bikini and spent the whole of the summer before I was due to give birth strutting around on the beach, belly proudly protruding. By the time my August baby came into the world, I had a deeply tanned belly for the first time in my life. Afterward, I threw away the pale-blue bikini. After all, I knew I'd never wear a bikini again.

THE FALL AFTER I TURN forty-five, the new rust-red bikini still hasn't been used, not once. But as if nature is trying to help me make the leap and bare my belly, the weather suddenly warms up again in mid-September, and the water is a pleasant 63 degrees Fahrenheit (17 degrees Celsius). I take a friend down to the jetty for a swim. It's early morning and the clouds have settled over the city like a light duvet; only a handful of people are planning a September dip. We're like the last roses in the flowerbed.

Quick as I can, I hunch down and pull my bikini on beneath my skirt and woolen underwear. Now my belly will get an airing, now it will be free! FREE! There's a notable lack of fanfare. While it's true I'm standing there in my bikini, this somehow doesn't feel like the major moment I'd pictured. Nothing really feels any different. I don't feel free—or unfree for that matter—perhaps more like a perfectly ordinary person in a perfectly ordinary bikini on a perfectly ordinary jetty on a September day. In other words, this is not an event worth striking up the band for.

For the sake of completeness, I post a picture of myself in my bikini on Instagram. That doesn't do anything for me either. But maybe *I'm* not the one that this picture is supposed to make feel different; maybe it's the people who look at me. It's a trend among women right now to show that they're brimming with self-confidence by posting naked or near-naked pictures of themselves online.

As Michelle Wolf quips on the subject of body positive activists, they're "being like, 'I don't care what you think about my body. I'm confident. Please like and subscribe.' And it feels anti-feminist to be like, 'Don't post that,' but at the same time, I don't know what our goal is here. I don't know what we're working toward . . . I think there's other ways to show that you're confident. Like, I don't think Ruth Bader Ginsburg's ever been like, 'I gotta get out of this robe and show people what I'm really about.'"

And she's right. Perhaps the question is being formulated all wrong. Perhaps setting my belly free isn't enough to free myself from my belly hate. I can choose to place my self-confidence in my belly and body or I can place it in my ability to think and write and be a good friend. Why should my appearance rather than my intellect set me free? I have to remember that. Next summer I must remind myself how thoroughly unspectacular it was to bare my belly.

WHO TELLS US WHO WE ARE? Who created the culture we live in? Who makes us define ourselves, our beauty, our strengths, what we do, what we are? All those times well-meaning relatives, kindergarten staff, and friends said "You look lovely" or "What a gorgeous dress"—is that what has made me obsess over what I look like rather than what I do? Why am I so much more gender than person? It really is time to turn the tables! Why do men I don't know ask if I'm pregnant? I have to shrug off my shame and ask myself how these men dare to poke me contentedly in the belly despite the risk of causing me embarrassment: Maybe the common denominator has something to do with *them*, not *me*.

All of them are involved with books or academia, but since that's where I grew up—in university circles, in libraries and bookshops—that's hardly surprising, is it? Could it be sheer coincidence? Even if it is, there's something I can explore here that is related to my belly hate. Something that goes all the way back to France in the 1640s.

In previous eras—I'm talking about two thousand years ago, in antiquity—people swore by *mens sana in corpore sano*, striving for a healthy mind in a healthy body. Back then the privileged were concerned about achieving a balance between body and soul, between physical activity and intellectual development. The thinker René Descartes ushered his readers into the modern age with *Meditations on First Philosophy*, published in Latin in 1641. The most important aspect of this book is the way Descartes establishes a watertight separation between body and mind. He is extremely concerned about distinguishing between what we can know about the world and what we cannot grasp, between mind and body. In other words, I can certainly say that Decartes' book was crucial for the film classic *The Matrix*: What if everything *only happens in our heads*? How can we know what is real?

I consider Descartes one of the main culprits for my belly hate. Why? Because of the dramatic distinction he makes between body and mind. What's more, he makes the mind as rational as possible, while the body is a kind of machine for carrying the head around. He also ranked minds based on their capacity for rationality, and perhaps it goes without saying that men topped the list. After that came women, children, and animals—and I imagine that, in those days, people with a darker skin tone would have ended up right down among the animals (this was, after all, in the middle of the age of imperialism and discovery, of slavery and exploitation). Descartes' ideas came to have a decisive influence on our collective relationship to our bodies because in Descartes' system, pain was associated with reason. Since women were considered more irrational than men, their pain wasn't as great. The pains women experienced in menstruation and birth were seen as purely mechanical processes, divorced from mind and reason. This approach to female pain was wholeheartedly backed up by the Bible, which explains it as Eve's well-deserved punishment for accepting the forbidden fruit in the Garden of Eden; for having *eaten too much* (an apple).

We know what many people and industries still think about animals' pain. According to Descartes and his followers, the Cartesians, children and animals did not feel pain because they lacked the rationality to perceive it. If they expressed pain, these were merely mechanical contractions. One thoroughly practical consequence of this is that babies and children used to undergo surgery entirely or almost entirely without anesthetic until late in the 1980s—yes, you read that right! That happened here, in modern, Western culture. The decisive turning point came in 1987, when the prestigious British medical journal *The Lancet* published a paper by Kanwaljeet Anand, which managed to prove that neonates experienced pain during heart surgery and should therefore receive anesthetic during the procedure.

I believe this does something to us, to the way we relate to other people's pain and our own bodies. Of course, I always hide the fact that I have period pains; I try to act as if everything's fine even as the blood seeps through my pale summer skirt during a meeting. As far as I'm concerned, period cramps have never been a good enough reason to stay off school or work, even though I've struggled with intense and sometimes crippling pain. I worked out that I've spent at least 450 days of my life suffering period pains. That adds up to more than most of the other ailments I've suffered—and the cramps tend to be a lot more painful too. But this isn't viewed as an illness.

Women's pain is, apparently, not scientifically interesting: female diseases have traditionally been less researched and assigned less research funding. A new report, issued as recently as 2018, confirms that this continues to be the case. And periods are not something we speak about at all; they are hidden away—a shameful reminder of our irrational and intrusive naturalness.

But if it's true that the body is simply a mechanical object, separate from the mind, we can mold and sculpt it as we wish: fill out the breasts, cut away the belly, lengthen the legs, break and reconstruct the nose, tighten the facial skin. None of this will have any consequences for the people we are; our thoughts will not change just because our bodies do. We are still living with the repercussions of the Cartesian conception of the body. We are surprised to find that depression can be influenced by bacterial cultures in our stomachs as well as processes in our brains, or to realize that the placenta lives an independent life, following its own will irrespective of our own. The belly is one of the greatest traitors in the female body. It affects our brains in so many and such unexpected ways, causing pain, mood swings, energy, magic. Of course it must be flat! To war against the traitor!

Academia is the environment where I have most often been asked whether I'm pregnant, by male academics. Even in the notoriously misogynistic film industry, the question almost never comes up. In university circles, it probably seemed logical to men to ask whether I was pregnant or wanted to have children soon. As far as they were concerned, I was and am more irrational than them, and the course of my life naturally leads me toward conception and birth. These male academics probably think that is my innermost, irrational motivation; they may perhaps guess that their conclusion is wrong, but this, at least, is how their words appear. I have heard PhD administrators sigh that women only apply for PhD programs so they can have children. Bear in mind that the alpha males with professorships have regularly helped themselves to young female students, semester after semester, without anyone lifting a finger (if #MeToo had hit the universities in the 1990s, there would have been a bloodbath). No wonder gender and genitals were constantly on their minds. My genitals were their business. They had the right to ask.

Stop Buying Clothes for a Future Me

SAY NO TO THE DRESS

I BUY TOO MANY CLOTHES. And it's all because of my belly. The first thing I think when I try on an item of clothing in the store is: How does my belly look in this? Can I pass as thin now? I suck my stomach in and twist and turn to make myself feel slender in the garment, and if it passes the test, it comes home with me. Soon after getting home, sometimes only a matter of hours later, or when I see a picture from the event I was dressing up for, I realize that this dress hasn't achieved the impossible either: It too has failed to make me several pounds thinner. I go up to the attic, furiously stuff the dress into one of the garbage sacks up there, and go out to buy a new one. I hardly ever buy an item that I end up loving and using. As a result, a steady stream of clothes is carried up those fateful stairs.

Only when, at last, I open the storage space in the attic to check what I have up there, rather than to simply discard yet another in the long series of garments, does it become clear that I am the happy owner of five large garbage bags full of clothes that are never used. After my latest weight increase, only a fraction of them even fit me.

I pick out nine items from the pile of clothes that have never been used, or have only been used once, and take pictures of them. This is my "wall of shame." I'm well aware that some of the richest people in the world run the big chain stores that push clothes. I know that some of the poorest people in the world sew these clothes. Why do I keep on buying clothes that I don't need, that are manufactured unethically, that also make repulsively rich people even richer— and that, on top of everything else, I never even use? I have to find out. Does my negative self-image make me easy prey for cynical clothing manufacturers who offer me soft, tempting solutions to my eternal problem? Is it our poor self-image that prompts us to fix and conceal, to dress up and divert attention away from everything we dislike about ourselves? Or is it stress? Some people think so. In a famous experiment, consumers were given the choice between fruit salad and chocolate cake. When they were placed under stress—having to learn a seven-figure number by heart—63 percent chose cake, versus 42 percent when they didn't have to perform the challenging task.

But I feel like there's more to shopping than that. Is this the human gathering instinct gone awry? When I walk into stores and surf shopping sites I feel a kind of relaxed peace: They're full of beautifully colored and textured objects that make no demands on me. Unlike everything else in life, which involves communicating, interpreting, expressing, and reading, clothes are just inanimate objects, tiny flashes of color in my "forest hikes" through the capital.

Neuropsychologist Peter Sterling thinks there's an explanation for everything from overeating to the climate crisis: Our brain is constructed in such a way that, when we lived closer to nature, we were supposed to be rewarded whenever we found unusual things that were beneficial to us. Maybe we'd find a bush of ripe raspberries or come across a squirrel we could kill and eat. When we find the tiny treasures that ensure survival, our brain receives a little shower of dopamine, the "reward hormone," and we feel happy and joyful. The same thing applies to another of the prerequisites for our survival: Our capacity to make the world even better and more fun to live in, our unruly, unrivaled creativity. When we use our creative abilities to solve problems and tasks, when we have our eureka moments, we will also experience a dopamine rush. Even when we solve completely trivial tasks, like identifying a hot-air balloon in a blurred photograph, our emotional center—the amygdala—is involved and anchors the experience in our memory. Eureka moments are fun and memorable, even when they can't be put to use. We love finding peculiar novel solutions, collecting up treasures and hiding them away, then putting all the things we found back together again, if only to form a new outfit. Our eagerness to collect seemingly useless objects that we can use in new and different ways is a fundamentally human instinct: We're all on a quest for a Chanel suit at a knockdown price; right around the next bend it could win us our fairytale ending.

When our work doesn't involve these sorts of surprises, which satisfy both our gathering and our problem-solving instincts, we turn our attention to the few raspberry bushes and squirrel trees available to us: clothing stores. Hence the hoarding. There in the fashion outlets, with their dim lighting and muted music, we find a whole heap of raspberries and squirrels all in one place. We—or at least I—gather them up and bring them home and stash them in sacks up in the attic. That also explains why it might suddenly occur to me to buy something that is identical to another garment I have in the wardrobe and already use: It's only natural to gather piles of things we can use in the future, especially when we know that they work in the present.

When the world was hit by the pandemic, we all discovered the irresistible power of this gathering instinct. We hoarded toilet paper and baked beans and canned spaghetti until the stores were empty. Before, we used to laugh at people who hoarded toilet paper and canned spaghetti; now we kept our ears to the ground, dashing off to stores that were rumored to have a few spare rolls of toilet paper left. Perhaps those of us with clothing collections up in our attics are just a bit more stressed and frightened than the rest of the world, who take it for granted that they have enough clothes to see them through tomorrow and the next year. Now that I've gone through all my clothes, I realize I've been planning for an imminent nuclear disaster: My animal-like gatherer self has ensured that I have enough clothes to last me the rest of my life.

ANOTHER HYPOTHESIS, which doesn't contradict the gatherer theory, is that all the clothes we buy ourselves reflect a desire to break free of the rationality and purposefulness that otherwise dominate our modern and efficient daily lives. I know that when I walk into clothing stores, I feel free. I get a secret and slightly sinful feeling of playing hooky. I've sneaked away from all the productive and useful tasks that I, as the mother of a young child, am expected to perform. Edward Bernays, nephew of Sigmund Freud and advertising guru, may well have been correct to speak about the irrational side of our shopping habits.

He was, after all, the man who succeeded in making cigarettes a symbol of female freedom by creating a—highly unhealthy—link between women's liberation and nicotine in several famous campaigns during the 1930s. By calling cigarettes "torches of freedom," he encouraged women to start smoking and even got them to associate cigarettes with suffrage. In my own era, buying a three-hundred-dollar dress may be an expression of the same liberation: Surely that must be the ultimate sign of independence—being able to spend vast sums of money on sheer personal adornment. It certainly proves that you don't have to rely on some man! Only a few generations back, my great-grandmother had to either sew and weave her own clothes—so it might have taken her months to get a new item of clothing—or she had to ask her husband for money so she could go into town and buy a new dress. Nowadays I, her great-granddaughter, can pop into the clothes store on a perfectly ordinary Tuesday and buy myself an expensive dress, just like that! *There's* women's liberation for you, right?

The irrational face of our shopping habits was also something Ernest Dichter wrote about in the 1960s: "You would be amazed to find how often we mislead ourselves, regardless of how smart we think we are, when we attempt to explain why we are behaving the way we do," he said in *The Strategy of Desire*, the book that helped revolutionize the advertising industry. I believe this describes my own clothes shopping. It seems almost impossible to put my finger on all of the idiotic desires that persuaded me to purchase the items in the attic, which I then never use. Freud spoke about the subconscious and all the covert longings it conceals. But I know that the only thing in my subconscious is five bags of unused clothes.

In an economics thesis produced at the Norwegian University of Science and Technology, authors Stine Anette Skaanes Berg and May-Elise Thunes Hordvik link daydreaming and clothes. They suggest that our clothes shopping is driven by our hopes about the future: Looking forward to the purchase and picturing how you'll look in the garment are at least as important as the clothes themselves. They also think that we buy new and different clothes in the belief that we can become completely different people when—at last—we look completely different. "This romantic relationship is an essential part of the experience," say the researchers.

Many of my clothes were bought for a future and completely different me. Do you remember being little and squeezing your biggest stuffed toy into the clothes of your smallest doll? That'll give you some idea how I look when I try on some of the clothes in the attic. They either fit me once or they'll fit me again in the future, but the common denominator is that none of them fit me *now*. They are colored by nostalgia linked to the past—the time when they fit me—or by dreams of the future—the time when

they will fit me. I picture dinner parties and celebra-
tions, sometimes the ceremony where I'm awarded
the Nobel Prize in Literature; I already know what
I'm going to wear by the way: after all, the dress is in
one of those five sacks in the attic!

One of the garments I've worn only once and that
I find lying crumpled in the attic storage space is a
bright green skirt by an expensive Danish designer.
At one time, I thought it was gorgeous. When I tried
it on, I felt so cool (I mean, bright green! What could
possibly go wrong? A color that hits you like a left
hook!). I was also convinced the skirt would really
work if I just held my stomach in absolutely all the
time, because if you're a supermodel with very long
legs and narrow hips, the skirt drapes itself beautifully around your legs. In fact, you only need to be
a person with a medium-flat belly for it to sit nicely.
But since the fabric was very thin and elastic, it was
also possible to walk around in this green sausage
skin when you were premenstrual and puffy, looking
exactly like a piping bag where the icing has coagu-
lated into a lump—I can't put it better than that. If
I'd had a completely flat stomach, that skirt would
have been absolutely perfect, but as things stand, the
bright green skirt is just a humiliating reminder that
I'm not flat-bellied.

The very jewel in the crown of my attic clothing
collection is simultaneously my greatest shame: a
rust-red dress by Italian luxury brand Marni, which

I simply call "the Dress of Shame." I had just been handed five hundred Canadian dollars. To this day I still don't understand why they paid touring authors with cash in Canada, but I'd gotten the money for taking part in a panel discussion during a book tour and it was burning a hole in my pocket. It could have been usefully spent on rent, kindergarten fees, or other sensible things. But I hadn't had a holiday that year, I was jet-lagged, and I'd been working sixty-hour weeks back-to-back even while on tour; I felt as if I deserved something nice—a reward! I'm just like Nora in Henrik Ibsen's drama *A Doll's House*, who hides macaroons around the house. She deserves them, of course, because she's the one who saved the family finances and rescued her husband from shame and disgrace. But it was a sad little medal, that secret macaroon. My reward, at any rate, would be extremely expensive—and designed in Italy, no less! I stumbled into a shopping mall in downtown Toronto where I found a store full of loads of famous brands: Isabel Marant, Chanel, Dries Van Noten. All the clothes in there were from previous seasons so the prices were dramatically discounted. My frontal lobe collapsed on the spot. I totally lost touch with reality, with the normal conventions of clothes and prices, with consequences and finances. It was as if I fell into a dark wormhole that transported me to some parallel universe where it was perfectly okay to spend fifteen hundred Canadian dollars on a dress.

The dress cost fifteen hundred DOLLARS before being reduced—as in "cheap," "a steal!" I walked zombie-like to the till and paid five hundred dollars for this asymmetric red dress in thick crepe that was "on sale" and even came with shiny buttons on one shoulder—gorgeous. An instant later I awoke from my shopping trance and was overwhelmed by a dark, implacable shame. Because on *my* body the dress does not hang loose, slightly asymmetrical, and cool; no, on me it looks more as if someone has stuffed a coffeepot into a handbag. IT DOESN'T SUIT ME! So I spent five hundred dollars on a "reward" that I haven't used a single time. Now and then I take out that red dress, try it on, hang it back up, and really *feel* the defeat, the shame, the financial irresponsibility. It still hasn't gone away. I've been doing it for four years now.

Buying clothes gives me a feeling of power. Having this money to spend on a dress means I have a bit more power in my little world. I can walk into a store as one person and walk out as another—a proper double agent! I can wear fifties chic, a figure-hugging dress, or loose bohemian clothing; I can be dark and mysterious or colorful and quirky. I enjoy changing my personality with my clothes. The very thing I find scary about my body—its changeability, the fact that it's constantly in motion—is fun when it comes to clothes. I feel as if I have a lot more power and control over clothes than I do over my own body. In *Face Value: The Hidden Ways Beauty Shapes Women's Lives* by Autumn Whitefield-Madrano, which deals with women and beauty standards, I discover that makeup shares something of this duality I ascribe to clothes: For many women, makeup is fun, it's color and beauty, and the esthetic aspect of it can boost their self-confidence. But for almost as many women, makeup is about concealing, hiding themselves, about shame and discomfort. A woman doesn't have just one reason to dress up but many, and there's a fine line between routine and obligation, between the feeling of creative energy and social anxiety.

While my clothes are certainly esthetic objects for me, I buy them just as much to change my body, to cover up my belly, or distract attention from it. I'm not bothered if a boob slips free or if people catch an occasional flash of my underwear, as long as no one sees that damn bulky, gross, absurd belly of mine: No clothes are designed to make people stick out in the middle.

WHEN OUR SEROTONIN LEVELS fall in the final week before menstruation, many of us have a desperate urge to eat chocolate. I'm no exception. But my cycle also has another effect: It makes me even more of a shopaholic. Consequently, around the twentieth day of every cycle, my husband will experience me at my most paradoxical: I stuff myself with chocolate, thereby expanding my waistline, while loudly bewailing the fact that I can't lose weight, and hunting for clothes that will make my belly look smaller. You may object that the solution is simply to drop both chocolate *and* clothes. I know that of course. But it's too simple. All I can do is try to control the waves of hormones with all the rational means at my disposal. I note down on the calendar: "Day 20: Shopping. Don't do it." Maybe I'll manage to stop myself if I know that low serotonin is what drives me from store to store. I stop going into town and that limits my shopping to some extent, but the internet has made shopping easy, far too easy. I buy an extremely expensive dress. It's useless and overpriced; it's pale-blue with a horse motif (even though my feelings about horses are ambivalent at best); it's a dress that is clearly designed for a golden-brown Brazilian model who's at least five foot nine, rather than a short author with a padding of fall flab. When it lands in my mailbox, I make a decision: It's time to put a stop to this. The shopping site in question has made it almost impossible to return clothes, but I refuse to be beaten. I communicate with one customer services employee in Hong Kong and another in India, which serves to remind me of the brutal face of global commercialism. But I continue to nag about the dress, whose terms of purchase included a fourteen-day return policy and the promise that it could transform me into a five-foot-nine Brazilian supermodel.

When, against all odds, I finally manage to return the dress, I'm seized with a burst of energy and post a bunch of my attic clothes on a classifieds site. But I only manage to sell one dress and end up *buying* used clothes instead. Admittedly that's more environmentally friendly than regular clothes shopping and doesn't put a single cent into the pockets of the mighty fashion moguls (who are, by the way, insanely wealthy: The man behind Zara, multi-billionaire Amancio Ortega, is one of the world's richest persons). But that wasn't what I'd intended to do. It takes 1,320 gallons of water to grow enough cotton for a pound of fabric and on top of that, there's the processing, the hours spent at sewing machines by underpaid women living under untenable conditions, plus transport and sale. That's no less true of the garment I buy through the classifieds site, just because it's passed through the hands of some other wretched shopaholic before reaching mine.

I think about the way I buy clothes to fix my own self-confidence, to satisfy an irrational need for liberation, *and* to get a reward. None of these are good enough justifications for mistreating the planet and my fellow humans. As I stand there with my bags of almost unused clothes, it strikes me that there's something really sad about constantly buying new outfits. These are garments that do not hold a single memory or story. I can listen to an album for months on end until the music colors everything I did in that period of my life. When I was a student, I only had a few items of clothing and whole years of my life were stored in their fabric like living memories. The pale-blue forties-style dress I'd inherited from my great-aunt? The days I spent studying medieval mysticism lie hidden in the pattern of the hand-sewn garment. A rather inelegant pair of crushed velvet pants was intimately linked to the British Renaissance. The clothes I owned in those days smelled of loneliness and doubt and pre-exam nerves and dreams of the future. But what about *these* clothes— the ones that are never used, or used only once? They aren't even time machines, portals to memories of my earlier life. They are nothing but guilty conscience and empty fantasies.

Forty years ago I read something in one of my favorite books and I must have forgotten it, even though I read it in my most formative years, when I was developing my own inner critic. "I should have remembered this," I think, as I read aloud to my own daughter one dark fall evening. How did I manage to forget this?

"What does that sign say?" asked Pippi.

She couldn't read all that well because she wouldn't go to school like the other children. "It says, 'Do you suffer from freckles?'" said Annika.

"Does it indeed?" said Pippi, deep in thought. "Well, a polite question deserves a polite answer. Come on, let's go in!"

She pushed open the door and stepped inside, closely followed by Tommy and Annika. A lady was standing behind the counter. Pippi walked straight up to her.

"No," she said firmly.

"What can I do for you?" asked the lady.

"No," Pippi said again.

"I don't understand what you mean," the lady said.

"No, I *don't* suffer from freckles," said Pippi.

Then the lady understood. And she took a close look at Pippi and burst out:

"But, you poor child, your entire face is covered in freckles!"

"Yes, it is," said Pippi. "But I don't suffer from them. I like them! Good morning!"

This is the beauty industry laid bare. It creates non-existent needs and manufactures standards that can earn it money. It hacks into my insecurities and dreams with products and clothes I don't need by promising that I can become a different person: But what if I, like Pippi Longstocking, say out loud that I like my body?

That's it: I'm declaring war! Death to the clothing industry! I must accept the body I have now! I must kiss goodbye to all the clothes that make me feel as if there's something wrong with me, as if I need to change my body and my life. There they lie, up in the attic, like a horde of demons that won't release me until I've settled my scores with them in earnest. "Why aren't you thinner?" they whisper. "Why don't you have longer legs?", "Can't you get yourself a swan-like neck?" There are dresses and sweaters and pants and skirts lying around in there, preparing to pounce on me with their malicious demands.

I decide to pull up these weeds by the roots, to get rid of the whole lot, not just one item at a time. Everything must go—now! My office becomes a clothing store and I post an ad on Facebook. I tell everyone on social media about all my bad shopping decisions and why I made them.

The more I tell people about the clothes and the irrational reasons why I brought them home with me, the more I realize that what I've wanted all along was to have a body other than the one I have; I've been hoping that exercise and calorie-counting would fix the problem, and that a transformation was immi-nent. It is not. It was not two years ago or five years ago—it is not now. I must open the cage and let those hissing demons fly out.

FRIENDS AND ACQUAINTANCES drift into my office for the clothes sale—people I've only met once, peo-ple I haven't seen for twenty years, some I only met a few days ago, and some I count among my best friends. They eat cookies, drink coffee, laugh and chat, and try on clothes. That's when it dawned on me: The changing room, where I have stood on my own so many times, twisting and turning in front of the mirror—I've always been *alone* in there. But today I was in the company of friends, old and new, and I hadn't given a second's thought to how I looked. The important thing was being together! All those lonely clothes would now adorn all my friends and acquaintances, and every single garment looked so lovely on these people I was fond of. I shut my eyes and tried to picture the entire city, with my friends wandering around it dressed in my clothes. Now we belonged to each other that little bit more.

Stop Dieting

SIXTY-ONE DIETS TOO MANY

WHY ARE THERE SO MANY DIETS if any one of them works? If there were one effective diet, we'd all just follow it and then get on happily with the rest of our lives. But that isn't what happens. The average British woman has tried dieting sixty-one times by the time she, like me, turns forty-five! And yet overweight and obesity numbers continue to climb in the Western world.

The first-ever diet book was written by Luigi Cornaro after he completely transformed his lifestyle, abandoning gluttony for healthy eating. And it appeared at the same time and in the same place as everything else that has shaped our modern world: Renaissance Italy. In his diet book, which came out in 1558, Cornaro wrote that he took care always to eat a little less than he felt like and that he decided what suited him best simply by *being mindful*. Fish disagreed with him, so he skipped it, whereas lamb caused no digestive problems, he noted. And, oddly enough—from our perspective—he writes about emotions in his diet book: "I have also preserved myself, as far as I have been able, from those other disorders from which it is more difficult to be exempt; I mean melancholy, hatred, and the other passions of the soul, which all appear greatly to affect the body." Cornaro, who grew up in Renaissance Venice, was grossly overweight and a heavy drinker by the time he was approaching forty, and that was when he decided to change his lifestyle. This was before the days of René Descartes, and it was natural for Cornaro to think like the Ancient Greeks: a healthy mind in a healthy body. Moreover, he lived in the country that produced the patron saint of dieting: Catherine of Siena had starved to death almost two hundred years previously, in 1380, thereby assuring herself saintly status. Several strands of medieval Christianity rewarded people for relinquishing earthly pleasures. Fanatics flagellated themselves, fasted, and gave away all their worldly possessions in the hope of earning religious enlightenment and an afterlife of heavenly bliss.

Being overweight has never been an ideal in our modern culture, and food is a site of great battles and absurd restrictions. Being overweight is pure, unadulterated shame. I often think with yearning of the days when I had a flat belly. But I am not made to have a flat belly, my genes speak for themselves. Nothing in my family history indicates that I should be tall and thin because I come from a long line of apples. I learned about this concept in a women's magazine I read back in my twenties, when I still bothered to buy them because I thought they were what you were supposed to read on the beach (it turns out I was wrong: You can read books on the beach and you'll feel a lot better). These magazines taught me that my body shape resembles an apple. There are also pears. Probably pineapples and bananas too. When I leaned up against my grandma's big, soft belly, I was leaning up against my own future. I guess I'll look like her when I'm eighty. My entire family is short and thick around the middle—a proper belly-family. We are short; we have bellies. We are apples.

While my height has remained absolutely unchanged since I was around sixteen, my weight has fluctuated by close to ninety pounds over the same period—that is nearly ninety pounds between my thinnest and gauntest, and my most overweight. The only constant has been my belly hate. In fact, I've never had more negative thoughts about my belly than when I was fifteen and genuinely underweight, with a BMI of 14 (the normal range is between 18.5 and 25). Even though I didn't have a belly I thought about my belly throughout my teens. My belly dictated my whole life. How it looked, what I put in it. There was one period when the only thing I would eat was a few slices of pickled beet a day (even now, the smell of it evokes a mixture of mild melancholy and slight nausea). Controlling my weight didn't make me happy, but that wasn't the point either. It wasn't happiness I was after. I think what I wanted was to harm myself.

In Norway, fifty-five thousand women between the ages of fifteen and forty-four have an eating disorder. Ten times more women (twenty-eight thousand) overeat than suffer anorexia, and binge-eating disorder is the world's most prevalent eating disorder. There are some recurring traits among those who develop eating disorders, such as obsessive-compulsive disorder and perfectionism, where no mistakes are permissible. Anxiety and depression are common. Your environment is also an important factor— whether, for example, you are surrounded by people who clearly express the idea that thin is best. One experiment involving mothers and their eight- to twelve-year-old daughters showed that when the women read a fashion magazine in front of their girls and made negative comments about bodies, their daughters immediately began displaying signs of disordered eating, whereas those in the control group did not. But that isn't how it was for me. When I was fifteen, I attended a school where I was surrounded by people who were almost militant in their refusal to care about beauty standards. So why my belly hate? And what happened afterward, transforming this unhealthily skinny girl into a forty-five-year-old woman with boobs, belly, and butt?

My body has never been biddable. Whereas I was stick-thin as a teenager, I wore an invisibility cloak all the way through from the end of my twenties to my mid-thirties. I could walk into a room and be invisible as air. I was ninety pounds heavier than I'd been when underweight, the extra padding distributed over exactly the same frame, and many of these pounds had settled on my belly. When it happened, I was in complete denial; I didn't see it myself. My weight just kept climbing. I didn't sit down with chocolate and potato chips with the intention of packing myself in a layer of fat. No, it wasn't that simple. Nothing is that simple with the body, with the way we use it, and the kinds of choices we make for it. Even tiny steps in a given direction can lead to becoming overweight. I remember standing on the scale at the age of sixteen. My weight was starting to head for a terrifyingly low number and it was then I made a conscious choice: When I saw that number, I decided to turn around. It must have been sheer luck that I reacted this way, because an awful lot of people don't; but I saw this number and realized I couldn't face descending further into that black hole. There was nothing more for me to find there.

Things were different when I became overweight. There was a very clear reason for it: I was sick and bedridden as a result of severe back pain. I had no job and, most importantly of all, I had no hope for the future. I was in my late twenties and thought I was on my way to becoming a young disabled person. As a result, I put on pound after pound over three years of terrible back pain and a sedentary indoor life. My belly grew enormous. My face changed. Framed in my huge moon face, my eyes became smaller, my mouth vanished into rolls of fat when I smiled. I comfort-ate, and almost never felt full.

The latest medical research shows that sugar is addictive, so once you've started to overeat unhealthy food containing sugar it's very difficult to stop. But I didn't just eat sugar, I also cooked my way through the culinary traditions of the entire world. I learned to cook Thai food, spent hours on Indian cuisine, rolled out fresh pasta in a variety of colors. I mastered Moroccan, Mexican, and French farmhouse cuisine and didn't give in until I banged my head against the brick wall of Chinese food (I find Chinese cooking really difficult). It was like a hobby and a frenzied fattening diet rolled into one. It might be the only thing I'd do over the course of a day: plan a meal, prepare it, eat it. When you have no hope, small things become so big. I ate because I was bored and because I was afraid of the future, and often because it tasted really good, and maybe also because I'd developed a kind of addiction to sugar and fat; I ate because I felt like a stranger in the world. I was always stuffed yet quickly built up an appetite again, and after all those years living an anorexic lifestyle, I was thoroughly sick of feeling hungry. I swilled down my self-loathing with a few glasses of wine and numbed my emotions with a delicious coq au vin and creamy saffron risotto.

> I lost myself
> My boundaries with rest of the world became fluid
> I felt so fat
> I *was* fat
> But not that fat
> My body didn't end with my skin
> I couldn't tell where the duvet began
> And the mattress was also me
> and the bathrobe on the floor
> and the baby-changing mat
> and the frozen food counter
> and the news about Syria
> They were me
> No wonder I felt fat

That's how it was, just like in this poem by Kristin Storrusten. Everything spilled over and I could no longer sense the boundaries of my body. And suddenly, one day, I found myself in the office of a slightly disheveled social services employee the same age as me, reviewing the steps I'd need to take to claim disability allowance. Enraged, I clenched my teeth. I decided I wouldn't go down this hole either. I have to get out, I thought.

I'm not wagging my finger here at all the people who have become disabled, because life affects us all in different places and different ways; but for me, it was like standing on the edge of a precipice and being given the choice: jump off or turn around and walk away from the cliff. I refused to jump.

Instead I started to send out job applications and, incredibly enough, I got a job. That changed everything. I began to work, full of eagerness and joy. I got to know new people and solved problems I'd never encountered before; food was no longer my main activity. I was no longer a massive stomach with arms and legs attached, I was a tiny but vital cog in the social machine. I had hope for the future. I didn't spend my entire time thinking about food. I started hiking in the forest and exercising; my weight plummeted and my pain became manageable. A healthy mind in a healthy body.

When I was thinking least about my weight, my body came closest to what I'd wished for: I reached just the right level of fitness and happiness. It's as if none of the really fun stuff in life happens when you're trying too hard, but only turns up when your mind is on other things: You rarely find a partner by desperately surfing Tinder; it's pretty hard to reach orgasm by thinking an awful lot about orgasms; and you don't generally come up with a fantastically funny idea by simply sitting down and squeezing your eyes shut. The best things in life don't happen when you most need them but when you've forgotten that they were what you wished for.

As the saying goes: "Life is what happens to you while you're busy making other plans." I think this is meant to be a melancholy acknowledgment that life passes us by. But I see it in a much more hopeful light: If I just make other plans, life will happen to me.

GETTING PREGNANT OPENED a whole new chapter in my life with my body: Hormones and breastfeeding and vitamin D deficiency and sleepless nights made me put on weight. Because my child wouldn't sleep. There are clear links between lack of sleep and being overweight. Numerous studies show that weight gain is a perfectly natural result of sleep deprivation. Subjects who hadn't had much sleep (4.5 hours) found that their appetite increased a lot more in the afternoon than those who had enjoyed a normal amount of sleep (seven to eight hours). Think about that next time you go to bed with your cellphone on the bedside table: The light it emits makes you sleep more lightly and if you spend a lot of time staring at screens during the day, that's very likely to affect your sleep and, by extension, your weight. Screen use at night is especially bad for our sleep. Before electric wiring filled every house with light, your home would have been bathed in gloom from the moment the sun went down, lit only by paraffin lamps or candles. In an ordinary rural community, people would go to bed at sunset. At five in the morning, they'd get up to do the milking. Before electricity and before the eternally pulsating light illuminated the great cities, nights used to be genuinely dark. You could go outside and see the stars shine like lit windows in a far distant house. Now the stars are outshone by the reflected light of our towns and cities, which is cast up into the sky; the light from Oslo extends nearly nine miles beyond the city itself.

The first municipal electricity generators were established in the 1880s. It is only a few generations since we slept deeply in completely dark houses, in completely dark cities. Taking control of the twenty-four-hour cycle, conquering the night, is a very recent innovation, which may provide a partial explanation for the wave of obesity in the Western world. We sit still gazing at screens, eat too much sugar and fat, lie around on our couches until we fall asleep in the weak glow from the smartphone next to us, and then sleep poorly and lightly. And we put on weight. It's hardly a mystery. What *is* a mystery is all the resultant hatred. Why is it, for example, that more men than women are overweight, but decidedly more women hate their bodies? Women are more often the ones who vanish into eating disorders and eternal diets, not men.

THE FIRST FEW YEARS AFTER the birth of my child, my weight went up and down in waves: I breastfed and lost weight, I slept badly and put it back on. Once the baby phase was over, I started dieting. *Of course*, I feel almost obliged to add. After all, I'd seen pictures of young social media influencers right after they'd had children. You were supposed to have a flat belly right after giving birth, weren't you? They did! What I kind of failed to take into account was that I'd almost never had a flat belly before getting pregnant, so why on earth would I have one afterward?

It seemed quite impossible to achieve a flat belly now. For many months after the birth, my belly was like a giant football that wouldn't deflate. It did shrink eventually, but flat? Nope. I downloaded a couple of apps onto my phone, one to count calories and another to count steps. In the intervening years, I've counted roughly 2.3 million calories on that app without managing to lose any weight whatsoever. I've counted around twelve million steps with my step-counter while continuing to gain weight. Why? Because I lack willpower, the will of iron that it takes to be a thin mother. And because I get manic. Suddenly, I see numbers everywhere. I count the steps to the bathroom and do an extra circuit of the storage space downstairs just to boost my step-count. And after I've completed my ten thousand steps, I feel like I deserve at least one KitKat. When the food is on the table, I don't see chicken vindaloo but 239 kcal per four-ounce portion—and I can eat twice as much of it if I skip breakfast the next day. I fiddled the numbers; I was the world's most creative accountant when it came to calorie-counting. And I thought about food absolutely all the time. I gave up.

My next dieting attempt involved trying to "fast" for twelve hours out of twenty-four—i.e. only eating within a twelve-hour window. This method has become very popular in recent years, along with the practice of fasting for entire days of the week, as in the 5:2 diet, for example. According to its advocates, fasting increases life expectancy. And that's true if you happen to be a mouse. In a lab. But I'm not. I ended up skipping breakfast and not eating anything until lunch. After thinking about food the whole morning, I ate a big lunch and an even bigger dinner. I gained weight. On top of that, I was furious most of the time. If I did end up having a longer life, it would be a longer life filled with rage. And what's the point of that? While I'm at it, what's the point of well-paid scientists wasting their precious time investigating whether breakfast is healthy or not? The results of this breakfast research are as yet unclear. Subjects who skip breakfast are less than a pound lighter on average than those who don't. Yet breakfast remains a hotly debated topic in dieting literature.

After that I tried the anti-inflammatory diet first advocated by US physician Andrew Weil twenty years ago, but all it did was make me profoundly unhappy. There were so many rules that I became discouraged. I found myself jumping at shadows: Anything could be potentially inflammatory—and you can *die* of inflammations, can't you? By now I'd put on even more pounds and was pretty dejected about my own body, which remained resolutely disobedient. In between, I'd tried a vegan diet—after seeing the documentary *The Game Changers*, which proves that top athletes' strength increased after eating avocado— but ate liver pâté on the sly. Of course, I'd attempted the obvious routes too, like dropping carbs entirely (try cutting out spaghetti with a five-year-old in the house!). Nothing has worked. I just end up weighing even more than before.

AS THE OBESITY CRISIS has intensified throughout the Western world, dieting books and apps and courses and methods have become a multi-billiondollar industry. In the United States, more than 170 million Americans are overweight or morbidly obese, and sixty-one billion dollars per year are spent on dieting. Forty-five million Americans go on diets every year. So I (along with many researchers) ask myself: If there are so many diets, why are we becoming more overweight? Do all these millions of people really lack any willpower whatsoever, or is there something wrong with the diets?

"Doctor?" Danish Nobel Prize nominee Karen Blixen is said to have spat out one time when playwright Arthur Miller asked which doctor had placed her on a diet consisting exclusively of oysters and champagne. "The doctors are horrified, but I love champagne and I love oysters and they agree with me," she said firmly, adding that she found it sad when oysters were out of season and she had to resort to asparagus instead. It's unusual enough to hear anyone talking about food in that way. But just consider the fact that it's so remarkable for a woman to talk about what she *feels like* eating and not what she *ought to* eat that this anecdote ended up in the history books.

Apparently, we always ought to eat ... little. Even though obesity is rising in the Western world, the beauty standard has not been adjusted—it remains just as skinny as ever. The fashion industry is colored by designers' dreams of the narrow-hipped boyish clotheshorse. Perhaps it's because designers want to do away with all that troublesome womanliness, or perhaps it's because all women, deep down, dream of getting back the body they had before puberty struck. Whatever the case, all clothes are seemingly supposed to look lovelier when draped around tall, thin people. It's as if we dream of being some kind of alien. The beauty standard calls for big, soulful eyes, and long thin bodies, a kind of pure spirituality reflected in the long limbs and triangular faces.

Perhaps we think about bodies the way people used to in the Middle Ages: Greed and laziness are still negative concepts, even though they've ceased to be deadly sins. One of the plus-size body activists I follow on Instagram wrote that she was reluctant to sit on a bench while waiting for the subway at seven in the morning. The reason? She doesn't want to seem lazy to the other people on the platform, knowing what they think about her body. It's possible that we in Western Europe also still adhere to the work ethic espoused by fervent Protestants in the nineteenth century. These religious groups believed that the only road to salvation was to work hard, all the time, without a break. *Then* perhaps God might show you some mercy. If you earned money, you weren't supposed to spend it on fun things like champagne and expensive dinners, but to reinvest it and keep on working. This ensured massive economic growth in Protestant countries. Max Weber called it the "Protestant iron cage," and thought—paradoxically enough—that it was one of the prerequisites for modern capitalism. For a Protestant, of course (whether a believer or not—the point here is not belief in God but the work culture that it created), fat symbolizes sheer laziness and greed, gluttony, and immorality. Based on this logic, staff who do not live an ascetic life in their free time too won't be especially attractive employees. In countless sectors of the economy, thin, sinewy marathon enthusiasts will always beat those with a bit of a belly and culinary knowledge from every corner of the world. Thin is efficient, pudgy is lazy. According to one study, people face more hiring bias as a result of being overweight than for their skin color or sexual orientation. Discrimination against the overweight is on the rise based on prejudices which assume that being overweight makes a person a lazy hedonist, weak and sickly.

Have you seen the film or read the story of *Babette's Feast*? Written by Karen Blixen—presumably while guzzling oysters and swilling them down with champagne—it is the story of a French cook who wins the lottery. For many years, she has worked for two sisters in Berlevåg, in the far north of Norway, and now she wants to celebrate her win by preparing a splendid feast for the sisters and the other people of Berlevåg—complete with quails and Russian caviar. The poor people eat without commenting on the food, having decided to pretend that this is a dull, ordinary dinner, because they are terribly God-fearing and don't want to appear gluttonous. So there they sit with the expensive champagne and the delicious dishes, pretending that everything is normal. Our entire culture could be seen as a Babette's feast. We eat better food and more of it, but we don't enjoy it. If Babette's feast happened today, one of the sisters would say, "How many calories are there in this turtle soup?" and the other would say, "I'm on a low-carb diet so I can't eat rum baba, but I'd love a spot of fruit salad—not too much, though, fruit is so hard on the digestive system." It's a sad life with far too little appetite. And it doesn't even make us any thinner, as evidenced by the continued rise in all the graphs of adult and child obesity.

When scientists were studying the reasons for this morbid obesity, they discovered something remarkable: You can actually predict who will become overweight based on their dieting history. People who have tried dieting risk becoming overweight. Ninety-seven percent of all those who diet regain all the weight they lost within three years, generally putting on a little bit extra on top. *Dieting doesn't work.* In fact dieting has such an adverse effect that reputable scientists have publicly warned against it: A healthy, happy, and slightly overweight person has nothing to gain from losing weight other than possible illness and stress.

I'M STILL WONDERING WHY my belly is the body part I most want to get rid of. Could I have hated my little finger instead? My chin? There's something utterly random about this body part I despise so much. Perhaps I'm suffering from body dysmorphic disorder (BDD). This is a serious condition and those who suffer from it are genuinely unwell, yet I would claim that we live in a dysmorphic culture, and that I am one of them. BDD is a condition where a person identifies a part of their body as "wrong" and spends a disproportionate amount of time correcting the "mistake." In order to think about the body in these terms you have to see it as a kind of construction kit, where various of the parts can be switched out. Or like a lump of modeling clay that can be molded at will. I've actually always thought that my body is precisely that, a thing I ought to be able to mold. The ability to alter our bodies is something we take for granted in our culture: What kind of a person am I if I don't shave my legs and my genitals, enlarge my small breasts, suck the excess fat out of my belly? I'm an esthetic abomination! I should at the very least squeeze myself into a pair of control-top pantyhose!

This collective outrage is not just a figment of my imagination. People who appear on social media with unshaven armpits or other body hair routinely receive threats or have their Instagram pictures blocked. Hair could provide enough material for a book all of its own, I find out: it, too, is a battle zone. When Julia Roberts waved to fans and revealed some serious armpit fuzz, it caused a scandal. Twenty-five-year-old freelance video journalist Ina Luna Gundersen received death threats after posting images of herself with body hair on social media— we're talking hairy legs here. A doctor I know was once contacted by a young man. He's worried. He's convinced he has a sick fetish. He gets turned on by women who haven't shaved off their pubic hair.

Failing to transform one's entire skin into a smooth, seemingly plastic surface is a sin, I've begun to realize, as I stand in the showers at the gym, in all my hairy, flabby glory, while young, clean-shaven girls with rigid upper lips and gravity-defying boobs regard me with skepticism. Like, why don't I take care of myself? It's one thing for me to be lazy and greedy enough to let both leg hair and belly grow, but quite another that I don't even try to do anything about it! After all, we know that body and mind are totally separate, thanks to René Descartes. Now it's all about having a beautiful body, and screw the mind if it gets in the way. I ought to be treating my appearance like an ongoing project!

"In the consumer package, there is one object finer, more precious and more dazzling than any other—and even more laden with connotations than the automobile, in spite of the fact that that encapsulates them all. That object is the BODY," wrote French sociologist Jean Baudrillard all the way back in 1970.

"The hygienic, dietetic, therapeutic cult which surrounds it, the obsession with youth, elegance, virility/femininity, treatments and regimes, and the sacrificial practices attaching to it all bear witness to the fact that the body has today become an *object of salvation*. It has literally taken over that ideological function from the soul," he continues, prophetically.

The body is the new soul. Being thin and beautiful brings you success in work and love; it can make you a star on the internet and on TV. Your exterior is your interior. Bret Easton Ellis' books *American Psycho* and *Glamorama* are about people who view one another as beautiful objects, and about the anxiety and violence that lurk beneath the slick surface. Because maintaining so much of a facade breeds anxiety. Those beautiful, well-groomed women who stare at my hairy, flabby form in the showers—maybe it's not scorn I see in their gaze but a mixture of envy and shock! My body is like a physical manifestation of Karen Blixen's devil-may-care response to Arthur Miller.

THE COMMON DENOMINATOR for those with body dysmorphia—among whom, I've now come to realize, I must in a way include myself—is that it doesn't help to correct the "mistake." According to the medical literature, wearing Kim Kardashian shapewear, dieting endlessly, or resorting to a plastic surgeon will only exacerbate the psychological problem. The beast is never satisfied; the more you feed it, the hungrier it gets. I've often considered visiting a plastic surgeon. But deep down, I know that liposuction and plastic surgery won't solve my problem. If I have liposuction, the fat will come back anyway if I don't change my lifestyle; it's like expecting to stop a river with a stone. And I can also picture myself so clearly ending up in the same black hole I found myself on the brink of when I stopped eating as a fifteen-year-old—how much is enough? When is the project finished? I can buy masses of clothes, I can exercise, count steps, count calories, stuff myself into Spanx, shave, and have surgery, liposuction, and filler. None of that will ever be enough, I'll never be finished; I'll simply end up becoming a body-hating seventy-year-old and then I'll die.

I actually think that the reason I focus my thoughts on my belly is to avoid thinking about other much more important things. It's safe there amid the belly button fluff. It's easier to focus on a body part that is "wrong" than it is to face our own mortality, fallibility, and vulnerability; the time that's slipping through our fingers, our death that is inching ever closer. Spare tires and tufts of hair seem easier to control than the overwhelming, incomprehensible chaos of the world. Of course, I don't believe for a second that they're thinking about death, those young girls who eat too little or those young boys who diet and train their way to six-packs. More and more men are suffering from eating disorders and muscle dysmorphia—the desire to have bigger muscles; boy children as young as six long for big muscles, I've learned from the research. That isn't what we wanted from equality. At the same time, we've been blinded by the gender perspective: Less than 1 percent of all research into eating disorders is devoted to boys and men, although the problem is on the rise. When you're young, perhaps control is what you focus on most of all, the desire for some kind of normality, regardless of gender.

But I *do* think about death. I look at my crow's-feet and the white strands concealed amid my mane of hair, and think about how I want to turn back time. I take out photos of myself at twenty. My face and gaze are so innocent, my skin so soft, life emanates from every cell and pore. Why didn't I understand back then how lovely I was, as all young people are? Why did I waste my precious time on hating my body? Why was I ashamed of my appearance?

"Every time I find an old photo of myself, I think how nice I look. But I didn't think that about myself at the time and I don't now, either, when I see new pictures of myself," says a friend, Anna. From a distance, I can see myself, too; I see my weaknesses and strengths much more clearly with hindsight. I remember all the self-loathing I nursed only five years back, when I'd just had a child—and of course my belly wasn't flat after the birth. But when I look at photos of myself from that time, all I see is a glowing and exhausted new mother. In five years' time when I look at pictures of myself as I am now, I'll see that there wasn't all that much to hate about myself now either, but by then it'll be too late; the moment will have passed. My goal must be to shrink the distance between the tenderness I will feel for myself in the future and the person I am now. I want to bring these two things in line with each other, so that I can look at myself in the mirror and think: "See how hard you're trying. You're really not doing so badly at all. You want some things, you're full of life and desires and dreams, you make an effort with your appearance, you smile—that's enough." Life is too short not to offer yourself what little self-love you can get. It's too short! What have I spent my time on if I add it all up? What have I expended my energy on? Did I use my calories on the right things?

I grieve for all the days I've spent hating my body. I grieve for all the time that has been lost. After all, the important thing is that I *have* a body at all, not how perfect it is. When I'm on my deathbed I won't regret not dieting more. I want to give more hugs, be kinder, read books, go on forest hikes, throw enormous parties where people fall in love with each other. *Those* are the things I'll regret if I don't do them.

ZOOM OUT INTO SPACE with me and look down at planet Earth shining blue in the light of the sun. Can you see yourself down there? No. We are so tiny and our time on Earth so brief. Just thirty thousand revolutions of this planet, that's roughly the journey we'll get if we live to be old, and then the whole wonderful adventure will be over. Am I supposed to spend my precious days and nights on our precious Earth on something as tiny and limited as my belly? Are you?

Give the Gorilla a Name

SEX, SELF-PITY, AND SEARING RAGE

I REALIZED IT THE MOMENT I came out of the railway station: My bike was gone. Although it wasn't worth much, my shiny blue no-frills refurb from the 1970s was a treasured possession, and lately I'd been cycling everywhere.

That's when I did something that surprised even me. I yelled.

"Prick!" I yelled.

I'd had bikes stolen before, but this was the first time I hadn't just turned around despondently and taken the bus home. Now I loudly vented my rage and disappointment.

My anger has many secret outlets. When I pick up the dirty socks my husband has dropped on the bedroom floor, I grit my teeth in fury. When I wipe the kitchen counter for the fifth time that day, I nibble away at a cookie or macaroon, swallowing hard to suppress my rage and frustration at being some kind of twenty-four-hour housemaid, without wages or decent workplace safety legislation. First I feel furious and then I feel sorry for myself. And what do people do when they feel sorry for themselves? They seek comfort. My own self-comfort sends my belly hate spiraling off in a vicious circle: 1) I eat cakes and chocolate; 2) I drink wine; 3) I buy clothes that are supposed to make me look thinner after eating cake and chocolate, and drinking wine.

I live in one of the richest countries in the world, where I have every opportunity on earth to achieve happiness and freedom. It seems ungrateful to waste my precious life brooding over a body part, I realize that. I'm ashamed of being ashamed of my belly. I should have better things to do. Above all, I should be spending my time making the world bigger for other people, not smaller for myself. Why, then, is my world so small that I direct my hatred and anger at my own body rather than at world leaders and general injustice?

When Nora in Henrik Ibsen's *A Doll's House* covertly snacks on macaroons, it earns her a teasing:

> Helmer: Hasn't Miss Sweet-Tooth been breaking rules in town today?

Nora: No; what makes you think that?

Helmer: Hasn't she paid a visit to the confectioner's?

Nora: No, I assure you, Torvald—

Helmer: Not been nibbling sweets?

Nora: No, certainly not.

Helmer: Not even taken a bite at a macaroon or two?

Nora: No, Torvald, I assure you really—

Helmer: There, there, of course I was only joking.

Nora: I should not think of going against your wishes.

This is how Ibsen describes a woman in 1879. Surely no man would speak to his wife that way today, yet I think the macaroons and jam (potato chips and a glass of red wine) are still just as great and guilty a secret now as in Nora's day. For want of other outlets for our lust and sin, anger and joy, the body and food become the tiny areas where we *do* have control. And if the only thing a woman has power over in life is what she puts in her mouth, there's a tiny scrap of autonomy to be had from dieting, and from monitoring and comparing other women's food intake with our own. Or perhaps just living through men or striving for affirmation from them. It's enough to make anyone pretty mad.

My imploding anger eats me up from the inside. I stand looking at myself in the mirror and gaze at the body that is the outcome of all the things I feel unable to choose or to do anything about. I grab my spare tire and pinch it as hard as I can. My fingers leave an impression on the skin. My belly, white and strange, looks like a sack of cold porridge. That's as far as my anger goes: to the fat on my belly, no further. Perhaps because it serves no apparent purpose. It isn't beautiful and smooth; very few men are turned on by this particular part of the female anatomy; and unlike my limbs, I can't use it to lift or carry or run or jump. It's in the way. It's surplus to requirements. It's in the wrong place. Why does my belly hate take up so much space in my life? What will happen to me when it's no longer an important part of my day?

IN A FAMOUS PSYCHOLOGICAL experiment about attention, subjects were told to watch a film. It's a very boring film, incidentally, but the viewers do their best to perform the task they've been assigned: to watch six people passing a basketball between them, and count how many passes they make. Half of the subjects don't notice when, a few minutes into the film, a man in a gorilla suit comes onto the basketball court, stops and beats his breast, then continues across the court and walks out of shot. They don't see it. This is how our attention works: We see only what we want to see, even when there's a gorilla slap-bang in the middle of the picture. So what is the gorilla in my life? If I stop focusing my attention on my belly, what will come into view?

Norwegian gender researcher Professor Harriet Bjerrum Nielsen discovered something unusual in her research. When children at daycare were asked to speak about themselves in sharing time, they were treated differently depending on their gender: The boys were asked open questions, but when it was the girls' turn to speak about themselves and their lives, they were asked closed questions. That's like the difference between asking, "Can you tell me in your own words…?" and "How old are you?" The first question creates space for an entire story, while the second has a single correct answer. Research into what we learn as children also reflects clear gender differences. When we take our children out on a forest hike, the things we point out and talk to them about vary according to gender. Girls learn general concepts, like "a pretty flower," "a tree," whereas boys learn species names. They get "sunflower" and "oak."

Why am I dragging child research into this when we were talking about belly hate, self-comfort, and Nora's macaroons? Well, it's because even this early on, a seed is sown that determines how we acquire power over the world and ourselves. I think this may be where it starts, the belly hate. Girls who aren't used to speaking up and telling stories about themselves have less power of definition. Girls get hung up on having the right answers and being smart, and end up doing well at school. But no matter how smart they are, girls are increasingly falling prey to depression and anxiety. And we now know that there's a connection between depression and negative body image.

I'm certain that we lose some power over ourselves if we are unable to speak about ourselves. It makes our world narrow, constricted. Stories, big and small, are an important way of drawing us out of depression and giving us power over our own lives. Now and then rote-learning may make sense, but I believe it can cause depression over the long term. My knowledge of memory research tells me that clinging on to the fantastic details of the world serves as a kind of antidote to depression, because depression robs us of detailed recollection, making memory abstract and gray. Sunflower is better than flower. The details are a kind of happy pill.

That's why I started taking photos on my phone. I take pictures of peculiar little things that make me happy: colors, light, flowers, or the little waterfall right by my home. Physician Torkil Færø has even written a book about how photography can help with depression—he calls the concept the "camera cure." After a while I stopped using my phone and simply looked. All those tiny details are what bind us to the world, by making it rich and vibrant.

Perhaps the big stories about what the world could be are just as important. All the big stories help us define ourselves and who we are in the world, where we belong. That makes our bellies less important.

Stories and literature don't just help us cope with anxiety and depression through bibliotherapy; they can also teach us more about ourselves and the inner lives of others. When someone tells you a detailed story, it fires the mirror neurons in your brain, as if you were the person walking through the room, or lifting your hand, or sniffing a flower, or writing a letter. These neurons, which scientists have been studying since the 1990s, fire when we think about performing an action and when we see others performing an action. That's part of the reason we yawn when other people do, or grimace in pain when we see pain depicted on a movie screen. By training our empathy, books and films—and all the other stories we are constantly exposed to—show us all kinds of ways of solving problems and understanding the world. For a brief moment, you are a different person. That makes the world expand beyond your own navel. If you own the world, your body won't become a battlefield.

ONE DAY, my daughter and I were on our way to school when she suddenly hugged my belly.

"Just think, Mom—there's a baby in your tummy!" Then she peered up at me apologetically.

"I'm only joking. You don't really look like you've got a baby in your tummy, honest," my six-year-old said to me.

I've never said a word to her about my belly hate; I've never stood in front of a mirror while she's in the room, and pulled in my belly or whined about not being as thin as I'd like. And yet she knew it. In everything from tiny gestures to implied words, I must have signaled to her what I think about protruding bellies. Of all the people who mirror me, this little person is the one who mirrors me more than anyone else in the whole wide world: my child. If I hate my body, I will pass that hatred on to her one way or another.

The world is so small for girls, but big for boys. Within the little cage formed by right answers and compliments about my appearance, by covert macaroons and suppressed rage, by depression and anxiety, and far too little contact with nature—within that little cage, I apparently live. What do I want for my child? I want her to think that the world is vast and marvelous and full of wonders and spiders and caring and carousels and morello cherries. I picture how she will be when she grows older, when she becomes a teenager, and I want the world to be a big place for her—bigger than mine, bigger than it was for me.

When I was fifteen, I found the world confusing and terrifying. I was a young person in search of myself, but I didn't have a fixed place, an anchor. Even my body was volatile and shifting and impossible to hold on to. I drifted from house to house, living more with friends than at home. Even the house of a grown man in my neighborhood seemed more enticing than my own. There I was plied with huge glasses of liquor, and there I was undressed and photographed, abused and humiliated—all the while believing this to be care and love. My body betrayed me back then. After that, I believe, I wanted to become a child again; I wanted to rid my body of all its womanliness—all the fat on my belly, backside, breasts, and thighs. I wanted to reverse my development, to stop growing to adulthood. Now I would have control. I had control over almost everything: every strand of hair, every calorie, every grade, over my body and my sexuality. I shaved my head, I got a nose piercing, I went around in big, baggy clothes. I read a lot and got straight As and I felt light—as if I had no body at all. It was truly delightful.

When San Diego physician Vincent Felitti was researching the causes of obesity, he discovered a remarkable fact: 55 percent of all his overweight interviewees had been victims of childhood sexual abuse on one or more occasions. He was right to notice this, given that "only" around 10 percent of women in the general population experience sexual abuse. Was there a connection? Several of those interviewed described how the layer of fat felt protective, like an invisibility cape; it generally enabled these women to feel shielded from attempted approaches by a potential rapist, or any man at all. They had built a kind of wall of flesh.

"Nutrition... has nothing to do with obesity. Teaching people about nutrition is essentially predicated on the assumption that people get fat because they don't know any better," says Felitti, after examining thousands of overweight patients. Because people *do* know better. After all, everyone knows that vegetables are healthier than potato chips, and fish is better than chocolate. Felitti's research resulted in a list of childhood traumas: If people can tick off six or more of them, they are 4600 percent more likely to become addicts as adults—and that means all kinds of addiction, from drugs to food. Because yes, you can be addicted to food. You use it like a drug.

Mind you, it's hardly surprising people develop a strained relationship with their body and food, since abuse can make you feel less in touch with your own body: You become a stranger to yourself and to your own needs. You become numb. It's important to remember that this doesn't mean that everyone who puts on weight is doing it to conceal sexual abuse. I don't even know whether that was true in my own case, or whether there were other reasons for me to become depressed and overweight; years of therapy have made it clear to me that there are vicious circles and virtuous circles, and when I'm in a vicious circle, I face not one but many gorillas.

But the research on rape and trauma does show that they alter your relationship with your body, generally triggering posttraumatic stress disorder. A large-scale study involving 1,600 participants—half of whom had experienced sexual abuse, while the other half served as controls—showed that rape influences self-image, body image, and sex life, and physical self-consciousness, as well as depression and anxiety. Though official statistics report that 22 percent of all Norwegian women have suffered rape, the real percentage is likely much higher. Like me, many will not have reported a sexual assault, whether or not it was committed by a person they know, by their husband, or by someone they themselves initiated sex with.

The fury I feel toward the man who abused me is vast and unwieldy. It was so much easier to direct it at myself, my own body, my own belly. But if I don't hate that innocent little bump, what am I supposed to hate instead? Am I truly supposed to direct my righteous indignation at those who deserve it? Am I supposed to become Uma Thurman in *Kill Bill*, the yellow-jumpsuit-clad avenger with a samurai sword on her back? That seems a lot scarier than tormenting myself. As I let go of my belly hate, my anger loses direction and no longer has a home. I just feel it warming the pit of my belly, like a smoldering log.

IN BENEDICT DE SPINOZA'S *Ethics*, first published in 1677, I find a curious definition of hate. "If a man has begun to hate a beloved thing, so that his love of it is altogether destroyed, he will for this very reason hate it more than he would have done if he had never loved it, and this hatred will be in greater proportion to his previous love." Does that mean I once loved my belly? If hate is inverted love, did I once love what I now hate? If so, it must have been before I started my period, before abuse, before stress, before depression and anxiety. It must have been before puberty.

This is the feeling of being a child: strutting about in a dress that fluttered around your legs, proud and happy. Skinny-dipping without shame. A body that was strong and happy. I was extraordinarily interested in what went into my belly—in a non-neurotic way. I thought a lot about candy and ice cream, and dreamed about the glass of soda I was allowed each Saturday. It felt a bit scary and a bit fantastic when I started to lose my baby teeth. I painted the world around me with myths and fairytales; everything felt full of mystery and secrets. To be six, the same age as my daughter is today, is to be crackling with energy, enthusiastic, bursting with life, in a body that is utterly out of control. I liked my belly, I can't remember any different, but no more than I liked any other part of my body. I remember how, in the summertime, I used to arch my back to push my belly out into the sun.

Is that how we see the protruding belly—as a symbol of childishness? It's as if, after childhood, we're no longer allowed to lean back happily, contentedly pushing out our tummies. I watch my six-year-old and think she is absolutely perfect, the whole of her body: Her belly sticks out when she's eaten a lot, just like a little chick that's gobbled down an outsized worm. The skin on her small belly conceals no secrets, no shame.

I have never loved my belly as much as I've hated it, so Spinoza is wrong. But there was a time, at least, when it wasn't the dark side of the moon, the shadowland. There was a time when it wasn't the one thing

I hated most in my life, the cause of all my troubles, shame, and repulsion embodied in rolls of flesh and fat. My belly betrayed me, not once, not just when I started my period, but many times, roughly 429 periods to date. It's a crime scene that causes excruciating cramps every twenty-fifth day; it's the place in my body where I've felt most pain. It's also the site of great magic because this is where the greatest miracle of humanity takes place: the creation of new life. I have to forgive my belly and let go now, try to let go of the hatred. I have to, for my child's sake, for my own sake.

What I wasn't prepared for was that this relinquishing would bring anger and grief. I grieve for everything that is lost, all the wasted time. I shouldn't have spent so much of my life hating my belly. Then comes the anger. If all that self-loathing I've carried around and focused on my stomach is no longer directed at me, where is it supposed to go? That takes me straight back to Hilde, aged fifteen: exploited, ashamed, frightened. That's when I first hated my belly. The abuse sent me floating out of my body; I could see myself from the outside, from above, as terror filled my entire being. My body was not my own. It was an object that could be used by others without my consent.

My body didn't become my own until I started yoga. My body didn't become my own until I had a child. My body must be won back every single day.

SO HERE'S THE QUESTION: When you stop hating your body, what reveals itself? Did your hatred of a body part simply absorb your attention, preventing you from understanding what really happened? What is it you're not seeing? What is the thing that eludes you? Where is the gorilla? What is its name?

Is it abuse? Is it the other defeats with which our lives are filled, and which have been obscured from view by that extremely concrete belly hate? Is it the world's injustices, which you alone can do nothing to change? And what about all the wonders the world is also filled with, which you are missing out on? There's certainly no doubt that when you focus so much energy on your own body, you miss out on an awful lot of things. Maybe even good things. When you let go, anything at all can happen.

Stress Less

BOOKS AND BACTERIA

THINGS I'VE DONE WHEN I'm stressed:

- Crashed my bike on flat terrain and gone flying over the handlebars, giving myself concussion in the process

- Forgotten my child's anorak and rubber boots on a rainy school day

- Forgotten that the table/chair/bed is where it always has been (many bruises later, I still don't remember when I'm stressed)

- Taken the wrong train to the wrong place

- Gained weight on my belly

The automatic responses of our bodies are largely controlled by two branches of our nervous system: the parasympathetic and the sympathetic. You're always in either one mode or the other because they don't tend to be activated simultaneously. When your sympathetic nervous system is activated, you're probably as far as you can get from being a sympathetic person, because you're really very stressed. When this part of our autonomic nervous system is running things, our body experiences a panic reaction, and the purpose of this is mainly to save our lives. Back when we were evolving into *Homo sapiens*, in close interplay with the nature around us, we might suddenly meet a dangerous animal, find ourselves surrounded by a forest fire, or encounter some other life-threatening situation. When we have an acute stress reaction it gives us a kind of tunnel vision: We hunt for quick fixes and definitely don't have any time to spare for daydreaming. According to the research, our brain becomes more like an animal's, flipping into "reptilian" mode, and we switch to primitive reflexes.

When we're stressed, our body stops doing all its regular maintenance work, which depresses our immune system and stops us feeling hungry. Short-term stress triggers production of corticotropin-releasing hormone, which suppresses the appetite. A really acute panic reaction may give us the urge to defecate, and our digestive system becomes drastically altered. Adrenalin, noradrenalin, and cortisol are all pumped out into the body, causing our responses to speed up, our pupils to dilate, and our heart to beat faster and harder, while our breathing becomes shallow and high in the throat. We are in fight-or-flight mode. This state is unsustainable over the long term, but for precisely the minutes or hours it takes us to extricate ourselves from mortal danger, we can cope with having an upset stomach or a less robust immune system.

The parasympathetic nervous system is more subdued but equally important. Whereas the sympathetic system is like a pushy, argumentative guy, the parasympathetic system is more like a meek, self-effacing suitor, who never turns up unannounced. The parasympathetic system is the one that deals with all the good stuff in life: wandering around in the forest sniffing flowers, cuddling cats, forming bonds of friendship, fooling around and laughing, telling tales around the campfire on a beautiful autumn night. Once our nervous system has calmed down, there's room for love, play, dance, and creative thinking. If you're relaxed and at peace, your digestive and immune systems will be in perfect working order and you can allow yourself to daydream freely—which is crucial not just for good mental health but also for any creative work.

The brain's "daydreaming mode," or default mode network (DMN) has many functions and may decisively influence how happy we are with ourselves. It isn't just a creative network, but a state in which we learn about ourselves and the world around us. This is where we anchor our memories (which can take several years to become fully consolidated) and this is where we plan the future. When we daydream, we pursue associations freely, without any plan or direction. The DMN is also the state in which "what if…" thoughts arise. And "what if…" thoughts are important for us. They mark the beginning of any creative process: a poem, a novel, a work of art, a piece of music, a scientific theory. The reason these kinds of thoughts are so important is that they make the world bigger and more extraordinary, expanding both our lives and our stories.

But what happens when we sit around glued to our cellphones? When peace and quiet and relaxation become scarce commodities? What if the stories we're constantly bombarded with tell us about bodies and appearance? What happens if we spend hours at a time gaming? What happens when everything we do is measured and weighed? When we count every mouthful we eat, and our high school exams determine our entire working life? When we're scared and stressed we operate more in the sympathetic nervous system—in the life-saving state of emergency. There may be a connection between how the DMN develops in the brains of children and young people, and the massive wave of anxiety and depression currently sweeping this segment of the population. And despite the efforts of Descartes and his disciples to convince us of the contrary over the past four hundred years, there certainly does seem to be some connection between mind and body, stress and overweight, depression and negative body image. A sick mind affects the body. *Mens sana in corpore sano.*

When Luigi Cornaro wrote the first-ever diet book, he was guided by perceptions about the body that dated back to antiquity. For people back then, good health required a balance between the four bodily humors: yellow and black bile, blood, and phlegm. If we had too much of any one humor, we would become sick in both mind and body, according to both Cornaro and the Ancient Greeks. Too much black bile would make you depressed, too much yellow bile would make you angry. And although the business of humors is sheer nonsense, it nonetheless strikes me that the octogenarian Italian's diet book may be the best one ever written.

Recall Cornaro's words: "I have also preserved myself, as far as I have been able, from those other disorders from which it is more difficult to be exempt; I mean melancholy, hatred, and the other passions of the soul, which all appear greatly to affect the body." How prescient that was. When modern nutritionists sing the praises of the Mediterranean diet—as they increasingly do—they seem to leave out the most important element. *How* do these people eat? I've sat by the warm glittering Mediterranean, in a tiny Italian village or on a beachside promenade in Greece, and eaten lunch surrounded by noisy families. They eat slowly, they eat together. They are *parasympathetic.*

ASHTANGA YOGA, the style I practice, is pretty hard, requiring you to sweat and stand on your head and lower yourself down into bridge pose. It draws inspiration from sources that include the traveling circus artists of India. You breathe deeply while doing difficult things, like tying yourself in knots or standing on one leg. Deep breathing is at the heart of yoga, and that's part of what got me hooked. Because breathing is one of the keys to the parasympathetic nervous system and genuine peace. Deep breathing calms the entire nervous system. Over the years I've been practicing yoga, I've learned to breathe deeply, right down into my lungs, even when I'm nervous or stressed. Even a single breath makes a huge difference, thanks to the vagus nerve, the "switch" that activates the parasympathetic system. It's called "vagus"—meaning the wanderer—because it passes through the entire body, including the neck. Laughing, breathing, and singing will all make you more parasympathetic and relaxed, more capable of daydreaming and creativity. Go on—give it a go! Try breathing deeply through your nose with your mouth closed and feel what happens in your body! Or how about giving just a tiny smile? Smiling triggers production of serotonin, the happiness hormone, no matter how artificial your smile is. There's an entire yoga style devoted solely to *laughter*. Founded by Indian physician Madan Kataria in 1995, laughter yoga has since spread to fifty-three countries and there are more than twenty thousand clubs worldwide. The underlying concept is that forced laughter very quickly becomes the real thing.

In my mid-thirties, I gradually established a routine of doing yoga five days a week before work. It left me buzzing with energy, relaxed, and ready to face the day's challenges. Everything in my life seemed to be heading in the right direction: I'd met a fantastic man (and didn't yet realize that I would one day find myself raging as I picked his socks up off the floor); I had a great, fulfilling job; I practiced yoga. I had a flat belly! I didn't spend the entire time thinking about what I was eating during this period, and without even noticing it, I started to eat healthier: more vegetables, less meat and sugar. Less alcohol, more fruit. My weight was stable and I was right in the middle of the BMI range that's considered healthy.

To illustrate the impact stress and sympathetic mode can have on you, let me fast-forward to five years later. I was forty-two and extremely unhappy. At this point, I hadn't eaten a decent meal for months. My weight had plummeted and I weighed a lot less than when I was doing yoga every day. I was most definitely not in the parasympathetic nervous system, but had instead been hounded into an extreme sympathetic response. I'd started a new job and was scared to death that I wasn't up to it. I spent every day in a state of fear. I'd stopped doing daycare drop-offs and pick-ups, leaving that to my husband. I worked instead of eating. I gradually dropped meetings with friends, alcohol, sleep, evenings in front of the TV with my husband, and reading books. I stopped doing all the things I enjoyed and spent the whole time working instead. Now I was thin as a pin. My hair started breaking and I had black rings under my eyes from sleep deprivation and anxiety. My clothes hung off me, which I saw as a welcome side effect. Now, at least, I looked like a model, a clotheshorse: a thin-skinned and thoroughly humorless clotheshorse. I didn't know then that this was only a temporary effect of a severe stress reaction. Over the short term, stress causes weight loss, which is hardly surprising considering that corticotropin-releasing hormone is an appetite suppressant. Only later did I realize that it also makes people less pleasant and flexible, less playful and creative, and less able to perceive the strange, fun, and fascinating details that make life worth living. My existence had become a black tunnel leading toward the inevitable depression, and I could see no way out. My new body didn't really bring me much joy, even though I believe I must then have been closer to my (imagined) ideal weight than at any other point in my adult life.

Luckily, all this passed when I resigned from the job. I decided to become a full-time freelance writer, which is also pretty stressful. Now, my body changed again. Because I'd been stressed and depressed for so long, I was prescribed a certain happy pill by my doctor that made me insanely hungry—on top of the appetite increase caused by the rocketing cortisol levels in my blood. I would eat one dinner for lunch and two dinners at dinnertime. I managed to pile on thirty pounds before dumping this happy pill, which had done nothing but increase my unhappiness.

This particular pill is not doled out because it guarantees good humor. Indeed, one of its most serious side effects is that it can make you feel suicidal. You also risk sleep problems, digestive difficulties, and depressed libido, along with everything else that makes life sad. This pill came about by chance, just like so many other types of medication. Take Viagra, for example: Initially developed as a treatment for high blood pressure, it just happened to have a very "fortunate" side effect. And something similar also happened with fluoxetine, the active substance in the "happy pill" known as Prozac. In the 1970s, it was found unsuitable for treating high blood pressure, psychosis, or overweight—the conditions for which it was originally trialed—but did temporarily lift patients out of mild depression, which made them more active (one of the problems with depression is that sufferers become so passive). The pill is enormously popular, and its popularity continues to grow steadily. Twelve percent of all Americans over the age of twelve take it. In 2019, more than twenty-seven million prescriptions were issued in the United States, to more than five million patients. In the same year, almost twice as many teenage girls as boys were prescribed antidepressants in the United States, 10.2 percent versus 5.3 percent. In 2022, the *New York Times* reported that between 2015 and 2019, prescriptions for antidepressants had risen 38 percent for teenagers compared with 15 percent for adults. The public health authorities are concerned.

Antidepressants like Prozac affect serotonin reuptake in the synapses, but since all of us have different brains that function in different ways it's difficult to know how such a pill will affect you in particular. However, the research clearly shows that the majority of people who take this kind of medication eventually relapse into their original depression. The truth is, there's no easy solution.

"Antidepressants rob people of their power. They make them feel as if they don't have any control and there's nothing they can do about it," research psychiatrist Joanna Moncrieff says. Journalist and author Johann Hari compares prescribing Prozac for depression to treating a broken bone with pain-killers: you still haven't treated the root cause of the pain or, to use a cliché, given people's lives meaning.

Prolonged stress leads to depression and over-weight, as my experience amply demonstrates. So what causes stress? In my case, it was the sense of being trapped in a situation. Life was lonely and joy-less, and the happy pill only made me more stressed and unhappy. I ate constantly because the pill made me hungry, and food was my only source of comfort. I ate because I was terrified of the future and lacked any hope. What I needed was life change, not a pill.

JUST AS THERE is a connection between dieting and being overweight, there is also a link between pro-longed stress and morbid obesity. Scientists discovered this after analyzing the hair of overweight people: They found that it was full of cortisol, the stress hor-mone. Prolonged, continuous stress triggers cortisol production and that in turn stimulates appetite. A 2017 study at University College London found a clear link between cortisol levels in the hair and BMI. The study involved 2,500 men and women, who were monitored for four years. The hair of those who were morbidly obese contained the highest levels of cortisol.

Stress has a variety of causes, but there are some obvious triggers in our society: All the research I've seen clearly indicates that constant stimulation and activation are harmful for us. If we are stressed and effective all the time, we are in a kind of hyperactive state that leaves us no time or space to daydream freely. Social media and smartphones are like a three-year-old constantly screaming for our atten-tion. The number of hours we spend on the internet is rising, work-related emails pour in on our phone at all hours of the day and night, and we do nothing to shield ourselves from any of this. And of course the global obesity pandemic is exacerbated by the fact that we've spent the past thirty years sitting motionless in front of a device that ensures we don't even need to get up to consult a dictionary. The interesting point here is that, as we work at our computers, we'll often be exposed to several stress factors during any given day—a deadline or a problem, an email from a dissatisfied client, a summons to an unpleasant meeting. And we have to resolve all these issues without having a chance to expel the adrenalin or cortisol that builds up in our body. If we were hauling timber, we'd sweat out the tunnel vision, anger, and fear triggered by a stressful situation by hauling even more timber. But now our stress lingers in our body, in our belly. And what happens to children who game for hours on end, playing out life-threatening situations on the screen? Prolonged stress also creates an inflammatory response in the body, which some researchers think may explain depression.

Roughly 39 percent of all the adults in the world are either overweight or morbidly obese, and so are a fifth of all children worldwide. Since 1850, the average BMI of eighteen-year-old men in the United States has risen slowly but surely from below 20 to close to 25 today. Poor-quality ready meals; easy access to sugar; a static life dominated by internet, TV, and driving; and a decline in physical labor are among the factors that have triggered this pandemic. The belly is a logical place to store extra fat, and, genetically speaking, it's an advantage to be able to store extra fat around the body, so that it can be burned in times of need. But belly fat is also indicative of something else: There's a link between the way our body fat is distributed and our mental state. Stress and depression are among the causes of belly fat, and ailments related to these conditions are among the most widespread public health problems facing the Western world. More than three hundred million people globally suffer depression, and the disorder is becoming increasingly common. According to Our World in Data, one in five people will experience it at some point in their life. A stressful life can lead to musculoskeletal disorders, depression, and rheumatic diseases, as well as burnout and loneliness.

DURING MY WORK on this book, I've spoken to many of those around me about how they relate to body and weight, body-shaming and self-love. Most tell a tale of shame and self-hatred. It's striking how many of the people I know have an unhealthy relationship with either food or body or both. While almost all of them could be categorized as some kind of bulimic, anorexic, orthorexic (healthy eating fanatic), or overeater, none of them has ever been formally diagnosed as such—simply because they view their condition as *normal*. It's so unexceptional that they haven't even considered seeking treatment for it. I'm starting to realize that this is woefully common, to the extent of being a public health issue: more than half of all women have a disordered relationship with food and weight, irrespective of their weight and age. It's hard to guess which of my girlfriends are concerned about keeping their weight down and which of them aren't remotely bothered—I can't tell by looking at them or guess their BMI. The shocking fact is that most of the women I know worry that their body ought to be different.

Two of my slimmest and most beautiful girl-friends stand out from the rest.

"I don't diet. I never have. I've never even considered it," Helene told me. The other friend was very much the same. Once during her twenties, she'd tried to control her food intake, but didn't like it and stopped at once. Both of them have opted out of worrying about their appearance and both look fantastic. They are well-dressed, well-groomed, and wear makeup, but they clearly don't focus much on their body shape. Some readers may object to aspects of this story. "But they looked fantastic just the way they were," you'll protest. "No wonder they didn't watch what they ate!" And: "Perhaps they have really good genes, unlike most of the rest of us." That's not true of course. We all have good genes, because if we didn't, we wouldn't be here; *you* wouldn't be here. An unbroken line of survival runs all the way from you to the first *Homo sapiens* two hundred thousand years ago—indeed, even further back: all the way back to the very first microorganisms that evolved from the primordial soup! Generation after generation of genetic winners survived the Black Death, war, cancer, cholera, and perilous childbirths—and here you stand!

Part of what has made humans the "winning" species on Earth—with all that this entails in the way of splendid civilizations and grim climate crisis—is that we are all so different. Some of us have really astonishing memories while others remember very little at all; skin and hair color span every shade; some people are practically inclined and others are highly intellectual and inventive; some build, and some dream and tell stories; some are tall and thin, while others are short and apple-shaped—and all this diversity has served us during our evolution. Difference brought us to where we are today.

Genetic perfection aside, the most striking thing about both of my non-dieting friends is their remarkably untroubled relationship with their own bodies; and, yes, I also believe they're fairly happy. *This*, I think, is how I want to be, far more than I want to have a flat belly. It's their outlook on life I want to imitate, not their bodies.

WHEN RESEARCHERS STUDIED factors that might explain the long life expectancy of strictly orthodox

Haredi Jews, they made an astonishing discovery. These people eat hideously unhealthy food that contains insane amounts of fat and sugar. Vegetables are almost entirely absent from their diet. They don't exercise. But they *do* look after each other! Their community is extremely close-knit (and pretty strict, admittedly—that's an aspect I don't envy). This also applies to a so-called "blue zone" region—a place with an unusually high average age—on the island of Okinawa, off Japan: There, too, communities are close-knit. They eat a fairly, but not excessively, healthy diet. More notably, however, the people in the villages of Okinawa sing karaoke together every week. Just imagine: You're well cared for, safe, and surrounded by friends. You sing with them. And song is, of course, one of the keys to the vagus nerve and achievement of a parasympathetic state.

Another key is gentle touch. When rats are stroked in different ways, the ones that are stroked gently at around one to two inches per second become much better at coping with stress than those that are not. The stress management center in the amygdala area of the brain functions better after this kind of physical contact.

Gently stroking the skin at one to two inches per second is, in a way, the "primordial caress"; it's the kind of gentle touch we automatically engage in when we hold a baby close to our bodies. It stimulates vital nerves known as C-tactile afferents, which are located on all the parts of our skin that are covered in invisible and visible hair (where our fur would be if we were monkeys). This touch is absolutely crucial to brain development when we are children, as well as to our ability to deal with stress. It also ensures that our brain develops a relationship with our body. You could say that this gentle caress is what glues mind and body together. The most fantastic thing of all is that these nerve fibers, which are so important to us, are located in places we ourselves cannot reach. On our backs for example. The fact is, our body is made to be stroked by others. And this stroking calms our entire nervous system. Considering what we now know about the effects of stress on our bodies, it goes without saying that this gentle physical contact is vital.

We also live in a culture where we often forget one crucial thing. Maybe we don't have the time and space we need for daydreaming, for becoming absorbed in our own thoughts, and for making up our own stories— stories that allow us to change the world. When we are depressed, our memory becomes very general, and our ability to envision the future becomes similarly vague: The things that make life so lovely, all those tiny details and dreams about life, are absent.

If we manage to eliminate stress, we may also get rid of a fair amount of excess weight. But more importantly, we may become a bit happier. If I stop brooding over my belly—which is, of course, a pretty stressful activity—maybe my belly will vanish. And if being happy and stress-free can result in a flat belly, that's a perfectly nice bonus. But if I had to choose between being unhappy and flat-bellied or happy with a muffin-top, I'd choose the latter—indeed, I *must* choose the latter. I need to find the keys to eliminating stress! If I stop being stressed, life will become pretty nice regardless of whether or not I have a bit of a belly. So I really only have two choices: stop stressing, sing karaoke with my pals, cuddle, and be happy, and maybe get a flatter belly as a result; or carry on stressing—about my belly among other things—and put on weight. Put like that, the choice no longer seems so hard. The important part is not the excess weight, anyway. It is being happy.

It may not be as tough as you'd think to find your way out of mild depression. When you read a book you're being purposeful and daydreaming at the same time: You go through the text with me, as I hold your hand and lead the way. Your thoughts wander yet you're simultaneously heading to a destination. You're interested in the world around you, but at the same time you have access to your own inner space. It's like going for a hike in the forest. Could I get rid of my belly if I only read enough books? I think not, but there *are* indications that reading can help lift us out of a mild depression, according to a field known as bibliotherapy that is particularly widespread in the United Kingdom. People have reported that reading books in the company of others has led to improvements in anxiety and depression. No long-term effects on depression have been proven but that hardly matters really. After all, it's never going to be enough to read just one book. We need many, many books and stories, many voices and viewpoints. If you read only one book, you only get one perspective.

But if reading a book is like going for a walk in the woods, what's it like to actually take a walk in the woods? In the Norwegian capital of Oslo, the life expectancy of people living on the east side is ten years lower than that of those living on the west side. The most obvious lifestyle difference between the two sides of the city is the relationship with nature: People in western Oslo hike regularly in the nearby forests. And, as researchers at the University of Michigan have found, spending just twenty to thirty minutes out in nature three times a week is a highly effective means of reducing stress hormones in the body from elevated to normal levels. Men also experience an increase in adiponectin, which helps protect against cardiovascular disease. Other studies have found that hiking in a natural environment diminishes stress more quickly than simply walking in urban districts: If you take a hike in the forest or an equally long hike in the city, your levels of the stress hormones adrenalin and cortisol will be measurably higher after the urban walk than the forest hike. But going for walks out in nature requires you to have energy to spare—which you won't have if you work too much, earn too little, and lack the time to do anything more than survive. When that's the case, it's easy to end up in a vicious circle, eating ready meals and spending your free time loafing in front of the TV—if you have any free time in the first place. The idea of getting outside and wandering around aimlessly in a forest is unthinkable if you're super stressed.

Research on forests has really taken off in recent years. While this may be especially true in Japan where people have been practicing *shinrin-yoku*— forest bathing—since the 1980s, a lot of research into the health-giving effects of nature has also been done elsewhere in the world. The slightly sad thing about this is that we shouldn't really need to do research into something that we know deep down is good for us. Yet this is where things are heading: Three generations ago the average eight-year-old in the United Kingdom would walk up to six miles a day through a natural or cultivated landscape, whereas contact with nature is almost non-existent for modern eight-year-olds, who are driven to and from school and various activities.

The late neurologist and author Oliver Sacks was firmly convinced that two things were good for our mental health: music and gardens. Both helped him to achieve peak creativity.

"In many cases, gardens and nature are more powerful than any medication," he wrote. Throughout his life, he would always visit the botanical gardens in the cities he traveled to, and he would often take his patients out into gardens when the opportunity arose.

Research shows that people who live or spend time in proximity to nature are less prone to depression. Access to nature has tremendous public health implications for the population as a whole. Sam Everington, a British doctor, has begun treating depression with gardening, and his program has spread across the United Kingdom. Depressed patients from low-income neighborhoods who tend the soil together become healthier thanks to the combination of community and working with plants. When a similar project was launched in Norway, gardening was found to be twice as effective as antidepressants. Digging around in the soil can also lift you out of depression if you happen to encounter a bacterium known as *Mycobacterium vaccae*. Studies show that *M. vaccae* has an anti-inflammatory effect on the brain—and inflammation is also linked to depression. In other words, there are bacteria out there that can make you happy!

HIKES AND EXPERIENCES out in nature can help combat depression, as can parks and gardens. What's more, going for hikes may not be so unlike writing a book or improvising jazz music. Your thoughts wander and your consciousness picks up on the things around you, not in a stressful or purposeful way, but more simply in an observant and somewhat aimless frame of mind.

Even so, hikes generally take place between two points: You hike from one place to another without feeling any stress, yet you have an aim in mind. I think about all the times I've roamed around the Botanical Gardens in Oslo and returned home the happier for it; and about the occasion I visited Virginia Woolf's garden in Sussex, which was just as overgrown and full of life as it was in her writing. Could it be that creative processes imitate nature? Research into the DMN shows that water plays a special role in daydreaming mode, as shown by a major research project in the United Kingdom, known as BlueHealth, which documented our relationship with nature, and its importance to our well-being and health. It found that proximity to water or the sea has a major impact on our mental health, and the researchers behind the project think that being close to the ocean makes it easier for us to activate the DMN. They asked twenty thousand smart-phone users to report when they experienced feelings of happiness in an app that tracked their location. A crystal-clear pattern emerged: Being by the sea came out on top—it's the happiest place we know of. After that come forests, fountains, and parks. Perhaps the reason is quite simply that we ourselves are nature and need to spend more time in contact with our original environment. Or perhaps we need to be in places where no one expects anything of us. The trees don't try to sell us anything or tell us anything. Insects and plants simply *are*.

IN RECENT YEARS there's been a boom in research into inflammation, such as chronic inflammation caused by stress. Scientists believe inflammations cause allergies and rheumatism, depression, overweight, and diabetes. Living an anti-inflammatory life—i.e., living in a way that prevents the development of harmful, low-grade inflammations—involves both reducing stress and eating food that doesn't trigger inflammation. If I sighed over the anti-inflammation cookbook earlier, it was because, like so many others, it triggered my sympathetic system: rules and pressure to perform invaded my life, even though the diet is supposed to be anti-inflammatory. Eating right will hardly help if you're doing it in a stressful way.

Stressing ourselves out in order to change can have major consequences. Stress is visible in our bodies all the way down to the cellular level. We age quicker. Our genes contain things known as telomeres, which help determine how long we are going to live, and prolonged stress can make them shorter, thereby also curtailing our lives. Stress really can kill us.

"The aim of this lifestyle is to achieve joy, balance, strength. Not an ascetic life regulated down to the tiniest detail that may make people feel virtuous as they post fantastic photos of gluten-free muffins on Insta, but lacks any joie de vivre or spontaneity," writes Swedish science journalist and author Maria Borelius, who has studied the latest research into inflammation, and the keys to living an anti-inflammatory life.

Her research reveals a startling fact: Sunsets can diminish the body's inflammation levels! The sense of being small in the face of nature may make us healthy and happy. Incredible as it may sound, this is what research into awe has shown us.

After everything I've learned about stress and bodies and overweight, I'm profoundly skeptical about the idea of making my body into an ongoing performance project, a place to show how virtuous I am. Every single diet is a lonely stress project and everything that causes me stress will only make me even more unhappy—and will even shorten the telomeres in my genes, as well as ensuring that I'll put on even more weight (remember the cortisol?). Who earns billions from our stress? Who benefits from making us believe that we need to look a particular way, that we must diet? Who earns even more billions when we comfort-shop chocolate and clothes after our diets fail? Books, clothes, courses, TV programs, clothes manufacturers—every step of the way, people are trying to monetize my poor self-confidence. Fuck the lot of them! I'll swagger around proudly with this stomach of mine—a great raging protest against capitalism!

I decide to stimulate my parasympathetic nervous system more often in my daily life: I want to be more playful. And what could be more parasympathetic than that? I go to the gym near my home and sign up for a dance class. I can't dance—not this style at least, not hip-hop and African and 1980s jazz dance. I stand right at the front beside the mirror, which is the only free spot. And although I'm no good at any of the exercises and my rhythm is totally messed up, I have fun; perhaps I have even more fun precisely *because* I'm so hopeless. If the dance teacher and the other people in the class don't like my terrible dancing style, who cares? This isn't a course for professionals. I look around and see young mums and older women from my neighborhood, and some of them smile back at me.

In the weeks that follow, I buy flower bulbs at a market in the Botanical Gardens and plant them in the chilly fall soil. The sensation of earth on my hands is delicious and as I picture how the garden will look next spring, I find myself looking forward to it. There's hope in planting flowers: hope that something beautiful will come after all the cold and all the darkness. I pretend I can sense the happiness-inducing bacteria beneath my nails. Bacteria are part of us; they live in our bellies and aid our digestion; they live deep within our cells in the form of mitochondria; bacteria live in our brains. We are 50 percent bacteria. Our bodies are nature, and need to be in touch with nature. Our bodies need to be in touch with other bodies. I hug my child as we sit by the flowerbed, even though she's covered in soil.

THE LAST BIG THING I decide to do is spend more time by the sea, which brings so many people so much peace and joy. My girlfriend Kristin takes me to the sauna boats that float on the fjord. As I sit there in the sauna looking out at the ice-cold water, I first become piping hot from head to toe. The flames lick at the window of the little stove and a calming crackle of burning wood wafts out into the sauna. The really expert bathers push up the temperature by stoking the stove with even more firewood and throwing water on the hot stones. It's hard to breathe, my face is flaming red, and the air burns in my nostrils.

Then we leave the sauna together, Kristin and I, and walk to the edge of the jetty. It's 52 degrees Fahrenheit (11 degrees Celsius) in the fjord. I slip down into the salt water with an undignified shriek as the steam rises from my shoulders and the morning sun gilds the islands that rise up from the sea. As I climb out of the water, the blood races around my body, and my heart beats hard and fast. I feel intensely happy and alive. And I haven't given my belly a single thought.

I Become Free, One Breath at a Time

STARS IN OUR EYES

ANY LIST OF THE MOST BEAUTIFUL WOMEN in history must surely include Shakespeare's Juliet, of *Romeo and Juliet* fame. So how is she described? Does she have a slender waist, is her butt big or small, are her boobs small or big? None of these physical attributes seem especially interesting to Romeo; for all I know, Juliet may have had a little pot belly. But Romeo appears to have been strangely fixated on a quite different part of her anatomy: her face.

> Two of the fairest stars in all the heaven,
> Having some business, do entreat her eyes
> To twinkle in their spheres till they return.
> What if her eyes were there, they in her head?

Juliet's eyes sparkle so brightly and beautifully that Romeo thinks that stars have taken their place.

I try to think about what matters to me when I meet a new person. Is it really the shape of their belly? Or their body at all? No, it's something else entirely. It's the way they move, their voice, their gaze. It's what we speak about, what we do. Above all, it's their eyes.

Neuroscientists recently made an extraordinary discovery: Eye contact has a thoroughly concrete significance for us. When we gaze into each other's eyes, our brainwaves synchronize. We look someone in the eye and literally "get in sync" with them. When I think about the people I love and appreciate, it's their eyes I think of, not their belly. I think about their sense of humor and intelligence, not about the clothes they wear, or whether their ass and upper arms wobble. What matters to me is how our lives are intertwined—through humor and conversations and experiences and birthday presents—not batwings and muffin-tops.

My child is fantastic to the very core of her being because of who she is, the way she moves, the life in her eyes, her smile. I tell her off and take care of her but it's when we gaze into each other's eyes in fits of laughter that something truly amazing happens: in our shared joy, we almost merge into one. The shape of her belly means nothing to me, as long as she's happy. Now more than before I try to view the people around me with the same love I feel when I look at her. I think: They were once children, they were once babies. Admittedly, it only works to a certain extent. I try to look at myself in the mirror the way I look at her, with an utterly unfeigned love and tenderness. It's unbelievably difficult.

WHEN I GO TO THE STORE for clementines, the front page of one of the tabloids once again nags at me to get rid of that "dangerous belly fat." When I check, I find that the Norwegian term for "belly fat" first appeared in 1978, before which it was never in use in Norway. Yet in the past nine months alone just one of the tabloids has managed to write ten whole front-page stories on belly fat. As recently as the mid-1990s, there were almost no articles on the subject in the Norwegian press, but by 2014, the number of articles on belly fat had peaked at 162. At the time of writing this book, it looked as if belly fat would clock up around a hundred articles, mostly in the tabloids. Belly fat sells, and we seem keen to read about it—in articles that present quick fixes for "the problem." None of the articles mention that belly fat is a perfectly natural result of our sedentary lifestyle, or that it might be better for us to love ourselves a bit more and stop stressing about our belly fat. Stress sells.

In 1884, the multitalented pharmaceutical entrepreneur Henry Solomon Wellcome invented a product he called the "tabloid"—medicine administered as a compact pill, rather than in powder or liquid form. His patented product would change the world. Nowadays we have pills for everything from pain and impotence to overweight and depression. An entire medical industry sprang up in the wake of Wellcome's fantastic invention, complete with laboratories and trials. Pills enabled us to resolve our health problems quickly and easily, and sometimes that's fine. But these days even *food* has become medicine! We seem to have forgotten that we humans are historically omnivores, who eat all kinds of things and generally mix it up a bit. Treatments based on a single foodstuff are now supposed to cure all our most complicated ills. If only we eat nothing but kale—or pineapples or avocadoes or even just meat—everything will turn out okay. One superfood can fix it all.

But it may be that some problems can only be resolved over time, like depression and eating disorders, PTSD caused by sexual assault, and poor body image. Pills are enticing and so are tabloid newspapers, with their diets and starvation cures. It's always all about speed: They sell quick solutions to difficult problems. Speedy can sometimes be good, but other times, a quick fix may prevent you from giving yourself the self-care you need, or trying to discover the more complex reasons why things got to be the way they are. Sometimes a hug may be what you really need, and that's one thing you can't sell as a quick fix. "Here's how to hug better!" is not an article you're ever going to find splashed across the front page of a major tabloid, even though it conveys an infinitely more important message than a news item about belly fat.

AFTER EVERYTHING I'VE GONE THROUGH with this book, after everything I've learned about stress and slimming, depression and anxiety, about childhood traumas, rape, assault, and period pains—why would I want to read yet another stress-inducing article about belly fat? I stand there looking at the damned newspaper, its headline about belly fat blazing out at me. Then I pick it up and turn it around, so only the back page is visible on the newsstand. I know it won't make any difference, but the mere fact of making this tiny gesture leaves me feeling a bit better. I realize now that it will take a long, long time to free myself from the depressive and dysmorphic belly hate that has taken up so much space in my life— aided and abetted by tabloid headlines and fashion designers, the slimming industry and influencers. It won't happen in the blink of an eye. Ditching a bad habit is supposed to take ninety days. According to many experts, three months of working on a positive change is what it takes to hammer home a new habit. For alcoholics attempting to achieve sobriety, every day is a new opportunity to conquer their addiction. In Alcoholics Anonymous, they work on a twenty-four-hour perspective: You can manage this for twenty-four hours. Then you reset the clock.

Every day, for the rest of your life. For me, a person who's channeled so much of her brainpower, so many hideous, negative thoughts, into hatred of her own body, it will take a long time to change my habit. But I can get through it twenty-four hours at a time, one breath at a time. I can try to create good days when I'll be kind to myself. I can do as Cornaro suggests in his sixteenth-century diet book: be mindful of what I eat and avoid melancholy.

I think about my child, who mirrors me. I think of all the other people around me who mirror me unconsciously, and whom I also mirror. If I'm constantly flagging my belly hate, I'll pass it on to those around me. I have a responsibility to them. I sustain them with my gaze, with my body. I am not alone, and this doesn't just mean that I must help those around me, but that they will also help me. Because we are all woven together by our gazes and our bodies, our stories and our dreams.

I DECIDE TO LEARN SOMETHING NEW about the world every day, so that my world will become bigger. Did you know that hermit beetles only live in one place in Norway—a cemetery in the southern town of Tønsberg—and that during mating season they emit a scent identical to the aroma of ripe peaches? Did you know that Leonardo da Vinci sketched a helicopter more than four hundred years before the first one was ever built? Did you know that up to 99 percent of the human body consists of just six elements: oxygen, carbon, hydrogen, nitrogen, calcium, and phosphorus, all of which were created during the Big Bang or in supernovas? So when Shakespeare wrote that Juliet's eyes were really stars, he was expressing a scientific truth! And now I've found out that I was born on the anniversary of the start of the French Revolution and that my name means "female warrior." These two facts are mere coincidence, of course, but still I wish to lead you in a revolution: "Long live love and cuddles!"— that must be our rallying cry: "Death to body hatred!"

I BUY A NEW BIKE. This time, it's a grass-green second-hand one, bright and shiny and freshly refurbished. I cycle down to the sea on it with Kristin, and we bathe together in the icy water that makes me sense my own outline. I take ownership of my body. I start doing morning yoga with my neighbor, which makes me feel alive and surrounded by friends, and I no longer think about my belly. I spend time with people who want good things, people I can do good things with— and *doing, together* is so much better than *being, alone*.

One afternoon, I decide to really relish the fact of being a privileged woman in the most privileged corner of the world who has bagged herself a beautiful old second-hand bike: I cycle right across town just to buy a loaf of sourdough. These days, I like to eat a light supper: a slice of sourdough toast spread with butter and marmalade. Instead of stuffing myself with candy in a guilt-ridden frenzy, I simply savor my bread down to the very last carbohydrate.

On my way back from the bakery, I stop in front of a bookstore. There's a sign outside that isn't trying to sell me anything, but is simply inscribed with a poem. Written by Nobel Prize winner Derek Walcott, it's called "Love After Love."

> The time will come
> when, with elation
> you will greet yourself arriving
> at your own door, in your own mirror
> and each will smile at the other's welcome,
>
> and say, sit here. Eat.
> You will love again the stranger who was
> your self.
> Give wine. Give bread. Give back your heart
> to itself, to the stranger who has loved you
>
> all your life, whom you ignored
> for another, who knows you by heart.
> Take down the love letters from the bookshelf,
> the photographs, the desperate notes,
> peel your own image from the mirror.
> Sit. Feast on your life.

I DON'T BELIEVE IN divine providence or mysterious connections. But right here, as I stand before this poem—with a fragrant sourdough loaf and a bottle of wine in my bag, with my struggle against the mirror and self-loathing like a searing imprint on my body—it feels as if this poem has been written just for me, just now, even though the poet died in 2017. "You will love again the stranger who was your self."

This has turned out to be a self-help book in the truest sense of the word. It has become a book that has helped me. Whether or not it helps the reader is another matter entirely. A belly book that ended up being about depression, anxiety, and sourdough bread, about bathing, cuddling, and dancing? That isn't the way I'd envisioned it. I've found out that billions of dollars vanish into the pockets of those who want to cure us of depression, clothe us, slim us down, tether us to the TV and the internet; those who write idiotic front-page headlines. Too many people are raped; too many suffer from a poor self-image and period pains; too many die in childbirth; too many can't sleep properly; too many are stressed and living joyless lives. I have also found out that I must play and fool around more often, and do delightful things with other people. What became of the poetry, what became of the very point of being human? Why do we no longer play? Dear reader, here are some slimming tips for you: Go sit on a swing. Take a walk in the forest. Dance as badly as you possibly can. Make a new friend and get them laughing. Remember: You have stars in your eyes and the world is so much bigger than your own navel.

Afterword

ARE YOU SUFFERING FROM severe depression or an
eating disorder and/or have you experienced violence and sexual assault? If so, I hope you will seek
help, talk with a friend or your physician, or book
an appointment with a psychologist. There are also
helplines available for those in need of immediate
advice and support. Many of the things I describe
in this book can help relieve mild depression—like
going for a forest hike, spending time with friends,
cutting out stress, making sure you eat a healthy and
varied diet, getting a proper night's sleep, and drinking only moderate amounts of alcohol. Most of all, I
hope you're taking care of yourself and that if you
aren't, the people around you are. I'm sending warm
thoughts to you, whoever you may be.

Acknowledgments

MANY THANKS TO Maja Lunde, who was absolutely
convinced that the little essay I wrote was a book, and
who persists in the steadfast belief that I'm a writer
even when I don't believe it myself. Many thanks to
Kristin Storrusten, who gave me a poem and showed
me the ice-cold sea and the boiling hot sauna at Bjør-
vika, and whose cheerleading and to-do lists helped
me get this book finished. Thanks to Peder Kjøs
and Helene Uri, who read the book, offering good
suggestions and ideas and amendments. Thanks to
Anna Fiske for all the lovely, fun hikes and evenings
spent together. Thanks to my consultant, therapist
Silje Fredheim. Thanks to my editor at Kagge, Guro
Solberg, who continued to believe in me firmly
throughout, and was such a wise and empathic and
thorough reader of my text. Thank you, dear Kaja
Rindal Bakkejord, for your thoughtful proofreading.
Thanks to everyone who turned up and took my
clothes demons off my hands, especially Elizabeth
Lovett, who even knitted a sweater for me—a fact
I'll never forget. Thanks to all the readers who get

in touch with me about my books: you're the reason I keep writing. Thanks to Ingvild Haugland and Cappelen Damm Agency for spreading my books out into the world, and to the wonderfully patient and compassionate Lucy Moffatt for translating my words so beautifully.

Thanks to my family for putting up with me. Thanks to my grandmother who taught me to love bellies and who lived with her "dangerous belly fat" until she was torn from us a month shy of her eighty-seventh birthday. Thanks to my child, who mirrors and inspires me.

Sources

Step One: Identify the Problem

p. 8 On social adaptation and the inner critic, temporal lobe, executive function, and DMN: Hilde Østby, *The Key to Creativity: The Science Behind Ideas and How Daydreaming Can Change the World*, trans. Matt Bagguley (Greystone, 2023).

p. 13 Article from Swedish teen magazine *Frida*, 1991: As well as advising readers to pull in their stomachs all the time and recommending lemon water ("the sour lemon helps shrink your stomach"), it also suggests massaging your stomach with circular movements when showering to get a flat belly.

p. 13 Never too old for eating disorders! Sixty percent of a thousand women aged sixty to seventy reported being dissatisfied with their bodies, while 80 percent controlled their food intake: Barbara Mangweth-Matzek et al., "Never Too Old for Eating Disorders or Body Dissatisfaction: A Community Study of Elderly Women," *International Journal of Eating Disorders* 39, no. 7 (2006): doi.org/10.1002/eat.20327.

p. 16 On how we learn, trauma memories, and cumulative memory: Hilde Østby and Ylva Østby, *Adventures in Memory: The Science and Secrets of Remembering and Forgetting*, trans. Marianne Lindvall (Greystone, 2018). See also *Handbook of Social Comparison: Theory and Research*, ed. Jerry Suls and Ladd Wheeler (Kluwer Academic/Plenum Publishers, 2000).

p. 16 On social hierarchies and how they affect our self-esteem: Nikhila Mahadevan et al., "Winners, Losers, Insiders, and Outsiders: Comparing Hierometer and Sociometer Theories of Self-Regard," *Frontiers in Psychology* 7 (2016): doi.org/10.3389/fpsyg.2016.00334.

p. 22   Golden Barbie: "What Is Golden Barbie?" Press—Redd Barna
        Ungdom, gullbarbie.no/what-is-golden-barbie/.

p. 22   Children are exposed to a lot of ads about bodies and
        dieting: "Nye tall fra Medietilsynet: Ungdom utsettes
        for store mengder reklame som kan bidra til kroppspress,"
        Medietilsynet (Norwegian Media Authority), September 15,
        2020, medietilsynet.no/nyheter/nyhetsarkiv/aktuelt-2020/
        nye-tall-fra-medietilsynet-ungdom-utsettes-for-store-mengder-
        reklame-som-kan-bidra-til-kroppspress/.

p. 22   Negative body image in different countries: Walid El Ansari and
        Gabriele Berg-Beckhoff, "Association of Health Status and Health
        Behaviors With Weight Satisfaction vs. Body Image Concern:
        Analysis of 5888 Undergraduates in Egypt, Palestine, and Finland,"
        Nutrients 11, no. 12 (2019): doi.org/10.3390/nu11122860.
        Here, the researchers write: "Independent of BMI, depressive
        symptoms were positively associated with body image concern
        across both genders in the three countries, and negatively associated
        weight satisfaction across both genders in Egypt and Finland. This
        agreed with a population survey in Switzerland where body weight
        dissatisfaction was associated with depression across the overall
        group, as well as in men and women, independent of BMI. Likewise,
        among Portuguese adolescents, body dissatisfaction contributed to
        depressive symptoms, without gender differences, and in the U.S.
        (2,139 adolescent males), boys with body weight distortions reported
        significantly more depressive symptoms than boys without body
        weight distortions. The links between body dissatisfaction and
        mental health are complex, with possible bidirectional associations.
        Postulated mechanisms include that body dissatisfaction stalks
        from an inappropriate highlighting of the importance of thinness
        and other unachievable beauty standards and, hence, may influence
        the onset of depression. On the other hand, body image-depression
        links are supported by neurobiological investigations, where
        hypothalamic pituitary-adrenal axis and serotonin system deficits
        are involved in mood disorders and in weight regulation, and brain
        areas involved in hedonic regulation may play a role for both body
        image and depression."

p. 23   On Jane Fonda: Melissa Romualdi, "Jane Fonda Opens Up About
        Her Decades-Long Struggle With Bulimia: 'I Assumed I Wouldn't
        Live Past 30,'" ET Canada, February 3, 2023, etcanada.com/
        news/965644/jane-fonda-opens-up-about-her-decades-long-
        struggle-with-bulimia-i-assumed-i-wouldnt-live-past-30/. See also
        Jane Fonda in Five Acts, dir. Susan Lacy (HBO, 2018).

p. 25   Boys and girls in kindergarten, open and closed questions, and appearance versus action: Karianne Munch-Ellingsen, "Gutter trenger også komplimenter," *Aftenposten*, aftenposten.no/norge/i/l1739/gutter-trenger-ogsaa-komplimenter; Trine Jonassen, "Den store forskjellen," Barnehage.no, September 22, 2014, barnehage.no/forskning-kjonnsroller-likestilling/den-store-forskjellen/114213.

p. 25   On boys' and girls' self-image and body image in school: Moria Golan et al., "Gender Related Differences in Response to 'In Favor of Myself' Wellness Program to Enhance Positive Self & Body Image Among Adolescents," *PLOS One* 9, no. 3 (2014): doi.org/10.1371/journal.pone.0091778.

Step Two: Know Your Enemy

p. 28   Periods: Christiane Northrup, "Wisdom of the Menstrual Cycle," DrNorthrup.com, updated February 6, 2007, drnorthrup.com/wisdom-of-menstrual-cycle/; see "Causes" in Kirsten Nunez, "Is It Normal to Gain Weight During Your Period?" Healthline, December 7, 2018, healthline.com/health/womens-health/weight-gain-during-period#causes; see "The Reason for That Monthly Heavy Feeling" in Whitney Akers, "Does a Uterus Really Double in Size During Menstruation?" Healthline, September 24, 2018, healthline.com/health-news/does-uterus-double-in-size-during-menstuation#The-reason-for-that-monthly-heavy-feeling-; Sabine Bott Pedersen, "Spør en forsker: Hvorfor får kvinner menstruasjon samtidig?" Forskning.no, September 26, 2016, forskning.no/spor-en-forsker-menneskekroppen/spor-en-forsker-hvorfor-far-kvinner-menstruasjon-samtidig/375094. Also on the uterus, see this article on copper IUDs and rising estrogen in the body: Mathilde Langevin, "The Uterus's Fight: My Findings on the Copper IUD," Medium, April 17, 2020, medium.com/musings-by-m/the-uteruss-fight-my-findings-on-the-copper-iud-74c2b1242fab.

p. 31   Hysteria: "Female Hysteria," Wikipedia, en.wikipedia.org/wiki/Female_hysteria.

p. 31   What happens in women's brains during the menstrual cycle? Quite a lot, according to these researchers: Zaria Gorvett, "How the Menstrual Cycle Changes Women's Brains—For Better," BBC Future, August 6, 2018, bbc.com/future/article/20180806-how-the-menstrual-cycle-changes-womens-brains-every-month.

p. 31   Michelle Wolf on periods, birth, and other fun stuff: "Michelle Wolf, *Nice Lady* (2017)—Full Transcript," *Scraps From the*

Loft, January 12, 2018, scrapsfromtheloft.com/2018/01/12/
michelle-wolf-nice-lady-2017-full-transcript/; "Michelle
Wolf, *Joke Show* (2019)—Full Transcript," *Scraps From the
Loft*, December 14, 2019, scrapsfromtheloft.com/2019/12/14/
michelle-wolf-joke-show-transcript/.

p. 34   How easy is it for fertilized eggs to attach to the uterus? Gavin E.
Jarvis, "Early Embryo Mortality in Natural Human Reproduction:
What the Data Say," *F1000Research* 5 (2016): doi.org/10.12688/
f1000research.8937.2.

p. 34   On the placenta: see "Possible Complications With the Placenta"
in Sara Lindberg, "What You Need to Know About the Placenta,"
Healthline, August 31, 2020, healthline.com/health/pregnancy/
when-does-the-placenta-form#complications.

p. 35   Hormonal production linked to menstruation and pregnancy:
Reshef Tal and Hugh S. Taylor, "Endocrinology of Pregnancy,"
Endotext.org, last updated March 18, 2021, ncbi.nlm.nih.gov/
books/NBK278962/.

p. 35   Research on why humans develop cancer has turned to the
placenta—because we humans have to be able to cope with the
placenta and the fetus acting like invaders in our body: Nicoletta
Lanese, "The Placenta 'Invades' the Uterus in the Same Way Cancer
Invades the Body," Live Science, November 17, 2019, livescience
.com/both-cancer-and-the-human-placenta-invade-tissue.html.

p. 35   The fetal cells are stem cells, which can travel around in the mother's
body reinforcing existing tissue, and even creating neurons, according
to research at Arizona State University: Richard Harth, "Fetal Cells
Influence Mom's Health During Pregnancy—And Long After," ASU
News, August 28, 2015, asunow.asu.edu/content/fetal-cells-influence-
moms-health-during-pregnancy-%E2%80%94-and-long-after; Robert
Martone, "Scientists Discover Children's Cells Living in Mothers'
Brains," *Scientific American*, December 4, 2012, scientificamerican.com/
article/scientists-discover-childrens-cells-living-in-mothers-brain/.
Y chromosomes were found in 63 percent of the brains of fifty-nine
women who had given birth to male children—the oldest woman
being ninety-four. That means these fetal cells can remain the
mother's body for the rest of her life. The reason scientists look
for Y chromosomes in women who have given birth is that women
only have X chromosomes. The Y chromosomes come from their
male children, who have both an X and a Y chromosome: Yasemin
Saplakoglu, "Why Does a Mother's Body Keep Some of Her Baby's
Cells After Birth?" Live Science, June 28, 2018, livescience.com/
62930-why-mom-keeps-baby-cells.html.

p. 36   This is how many mothers die in childbirth worldwide: "Svangerskapsrelatert dødelighet," FN-Sambandet (United Nations Association of Norway), fn.no/Statistikk/moedredoedelighet. This is how many mothers die in childbirth in Norway: Elisabeth Lofthus, "Fødsel: Fem mødre dør hvert år i Norge," *Dagbladet*, May 5, 2014, dagbladet.no/tema/fodsel-fem-modre-dor-hvert-ar-i-norge/61334521.

p. 36   Pelvis size versus the child's head: Markus Lindholm, *Evolusjon: Naturens kulturhistorie* (Spartacus, 2012).

p. 40   René Descartes: *Meditations on First Philosophy*, trans. John Cottingham (Cambridge University Press, 2017).

p. 41   Egil A. Fors on pain and pain relief: See Fors' chapter in the anthology *Blod og bein—lidelse, lindring og behandling i norsk medisinhistorie* (Nasjonalbiblioteket, 2019).

p. 42   To this day, less research is done on diseases that affect women than on those that affect men: Anne Winsnes Rødland, *Hva vet vi om kvinners helse? Rapport fra forprosjektet til kvinnehelseportalen .no*, April 2018, kjonnsforskning.no/sites/default/files/rapporter/ kvinnehelserapport_final_150518_med_isbn.pdf.

Step Three: Stop Buying Clothes for a Future Me

p. 46   Seven explanations for irrational shopping: Alain Samson, "Seven Reasons Why We're Irrational Shoppers," Psychology Today, September 25, 2013, psychologytoday.com/us/blog/ consumed/201309/seven-reasons-why-were-irrational-shoppers.

p. 47   Peter Sterling: *What Is Health? Allostasis and the Evolution of Human Design* (MIT Press, 2020).

p. 49   On Edward Bernays and the spectacular work he did for Lucky Strike, which changed the course of advertising history: Rakhi Chakraborty, "Torches of Freedom: How The World's First PR Campaign Came to Be," YourStory.com, August 6, 2014, yourstory .com/2014/08/torches-of-freedom.

p. 50   On Ernest Dichter: "Retail Therapy," *The Economist*, December 17, 2011, economist.com/christmas-specials/2011/12/17/retail-therapy.

p. 51   NTNU thesis on shopping: Stine Anette Skaanes Berg and May-Elise Thunes Hordvik, "Daydreaming & Consumption: A Greater Pleasure to Chase Than to Possess," NTNU Trondheim Business School, master's thesis, May 24, 2018, ntnuopen.ntnu.no/ntnu-xmlui/bitstream/handle/11250/2577652/Berg%20og%20Hordvik .pdf?sequence=1&isAllowed=y.

p. 55   Autumn Whitefield-Madrano: *Face Value: The Hidden Ways Beauty Shapes Women's Lives* (Simon & Schuster, 2017).

p. 57   The founder of Zara is featured on the Forbes Billionaires List; he's amassed a fortune worth roughly $85 billion: Avery Hartmans, "Meet Amancio Ortega, the Fiercely Private Zara Founder Who Built a $77 Billion Fast-Fashion Empire," Business Insider, updated March 28, 2023, businessinsider.com/zara-founder-amancio-ortegas-life-and-houses?r=us&ir=t.

p. 57   Cotton production: "un Helps Fashion Industry Shift to Low Carbon," United Nations Climate Change, September 6, 2018, unfccc.int/news/un-helps-fashion-industry-shift-to-low-carbon.

p. 58   Pippi Longstocking on freckles: Astrid Lindgren, *Pippi Goes On Board*, trans. Susan Beard (Viking, 2020).

Step Four: Stop Dieting

p. 62   British women try two diets a year from the age of sixteen: "Women Have Tried 61 Diets by the Age of 45 in the Constant Battle to Stay Slim," *Daily Mail*, updated March 20, 2012, dailymail.co.uk/health/article-2117445/Women-tried-61-diets-age-45-constant-battle-stay-slim.html.

p. 62   Forty percent of us have tried to lose weight in the past five years: Yet, slowly but surely, the population continues to gain weight. How can this add up, if dieting really works? Dieting doesn't work. See Philippe Jacquet et al., "How Dieting Might Make Some Fatter: Modeling Weight Cycling Toward Obesity From a Perspective of Body Composition Autoregulation," *Nature* 44 (2020): doi.org/10.1038/s41366-020-0547-1.

p. 62   Cornaro's diet book: Conor Heffernan, "Diet Advice From the 16th Century," Physical Culture Study, November 12, 2015, physicalculturestudy.com/2015/11/12/diet-advice-from-the-16th-century; "The History of Dieting," Skyterra, skyterrawellness.com/history-of-dieting/. You can read the entire diet book in English here: Luigi Cornaro, *The Art of Long Living* (William F. Butler, 1917), archive.org/details/artoflivinglong00corniala.

p. 65   On eating disorders: see Elin Skretting Lunde et al., *Kvinners liv og helse siste 20 år*, Statistisk sentralbyrå (Statistics Norway), September 27, 2022, ssb.no/helse/helsetjenester/artikler/kvinners-liv-og-helse-siste-20-ar/_/attachment/inline/c631d917-23e0-4f6d-aeaf-adc41747c6dc:f888278b9158f6df00294ec20c14 41dbe7baf661/RAPP2022-41.pdf, page 41; Silje Førsund, "Anoreksi:

Disse jentene får spiseforstyrrelser," κκ, updated June 29, 2017, kk.no/livstil/disse-jentene-far-spiseforstyrrelser/67899049. See also patient, journalist, and nurse Ingeborg Senneset's *Anorektisk* (Cappelen Damm, 2017).

p. 65   On anorexia and anxiety: Florian Junne et al., "The Relationship of Body Image With Symptoms of Depression and Anxiety in Patients With Anorexia Nervosa During Outpatient Psychotherapy: Results of the ANTOP Study," *Psychotherapy Theory Research Practice Training* 53, no. 2 (2016): doi.org/10.1037/pst0000064; "Anorexia Nervosa," Mental Health Foundation, mentalhealth.org.uk/a-to-z/a/anorexia-nervosa; Tammy Beasley, "How Intermittent Fasting (IF) and Eating Disorders Are Similar," Alsana, alsana.com/intermittent-fasting-if-resembles-eating-disorder-behavior/.

p. 65   The study about mothers, daughters, and fashion magazines: Charlotte M. Handford et al., "The Influence of Maternal Modeling on Body Image Concerns and Eating Disturbances in Preadolescent Girls," *Behaviour Research and Therapy* 100 (2018): doi.org/10.1016/j.brat.2017.11.001.

p. 68   Kristin Storrusten: *Barsel* (Tiden, 2017).

p. 70   Sleep deprivation affects weight: Tianna Hicklin, "Molecular Ties Between Lack of Sleep and Weight Gain," National Institutes of Health, March 22, 2016, nih.gov/news-events/nih-research-matters/molecular-ties-between-lack-sleep-weight-gain.

p. 70   On sleeping with light vs. in darkness: Sigri Sandberg, *An Ode to Darkness*, trans. Siân Mackie (Sphere, 2019).

p. 71   On obesity in the West, see, for example, the percentages of overweight men and women in Norway: Haakon Eduard Meyer et al., "Overweight and Obesity in Norway," Norwegian Institute of Public Health, updated March 11, 2017, fhi.no/en/op/hin/health-disease/overweight-and-obesity-in-norway---/.

p. 73   About fasting: Maria Borelius, *Health Revolution: Finding Happiness and Health Through an Anti-Inflammatory Lifestyle*, trans. Sonia Wichmann (Harper Design, 2019). The research on breakfast and dieting is unclear: we can't be sure that eating breakfast is as healthy as many scientists claim, but neither can we be certain that it's a particularly good idea to skip breakfast. I say fuck the research—just go ahead and eat breakfast if you feel like eating breakfast. Perhaps these particular scientists could do with finding something else to spend their time on. See also "The Quality of Evidence Is Low" in Heather Grey, "Should You Eat Breakfast If You Want to Lose Weight? Here's What to Know," Healthline,

February 11, 2019, healthline.com/health-news/is-breakfast-good-or-bad-for-weightloss#The-quality-of-evidence-is-low.

p. 74 Documentary on the vegan diet: *The Game Changers*, dir. Louie Psihoyos (Netflix, 2018).

p. 74 On obesity: For worldwide obesity, see "Obesity," World Health Organization, who.int/health-topics/obesity#tab=tab_1; for obesity in the United States, see Christopher J.L. Murray et al., "The Vast Majority of American Adults Are Overweight or Obese, and Weight Is a Growing Problem Among US Children," Institute for Health Metrics and Evaluation, May 28, 2014, healthdata.org/news-release/vast-majority-american-adults-are-overweight-or-obese-and-weight-growing-problem-among; for obesity in Norway, see Joachim Wettergreen, "Vi er kanskje ikke så overvektige likevel?" Statistics Norway, January 16, 2017, ssb.no/helse/artikler-og-publikasjoner/vi-er-kanskje-ikke-sa-overvektige-likevel.

p. 74 Karen Blixen's diet, and the lunch with Arthur Miller and Marilyn Monroe: Eve Goldberg, "Lunch With Carson," *The Rumpus*, July 15, 2010, therumpus.net/2010/07/lunch-with-carson/.

p. 76 Max Weber: *The Protestant Ethic and the Spirit of Capitalism*, trans. Talcott Parsons (Unwin, 1965).

p. 76 People work more in Protestant countries: Ingrid Spilde, "Protestanter jobber mer," Forskning.no, December 24, 2007, forskning.no/arbeid-religion/protestanter-jobber-mer/993174.

p. 76 Overweight people face increasing discrimination; they are assumed to be lazy and unhealthy: Janice Gassam Asare, "The Discrimination No One Talks About: Weight Discrimination," *Forbes*, January 31, 2019, forbes.com/sites/janicegassam/2019/01/31/the-discrimination-no-one-talks-about-weight-discrimination/?sh=2b88ecdf3e5f; "Weight Revealed as the UK's Most Common Form of Discrimination," British Liver Trust, October 11, 2018, britishlivertrust.org.uk/weight-uks-most-common-discrimination/; Susie Orbach, "Britain's Obesity Strategy Ignores the Science: Dieting Doesn't Work," *The Guardian*, July 28, 2020, theguardian.com/commentisfree/2020/jul/28/britain-obesity-strategy-ignore-science-dieting-calories-stigmatising-fat. In the United Kingdom, overweight is a more common cause of discrimination than sexual orientation or skin color: Edith Tollschein, "Weight Bias in Hiring," Medium, July 15, 2019, medium.com/swlh/weight-bias-in-hiring-77aeab0d1f9d.

p. 76 Recruiting procedures discriminate against overweight people: Stuart W. Flint et al., "Obesity Discrimination in the Recruitment

Process: 'You're Not Hired!'" *Frontiers in Psychology* 7 (2016): doi.org/10.3389/fpsyg.2016.00647; Ronald Alsop, "Fat People Earn Less and Have a Harder Time Finding Work," BBC Worklife, December 1, 2016, bbc.com/worklife/article/20161130-fat-people-earn-less-and-have-a-harder-time-finding-work.

p. 77   Karen Blixen: *Babette's Feast and Other Stories* (Penguin Classics, 2013).

p. 78   Want to predict overweight? Look at a person's dieting history. A person who has dieted is more likely to become overweight: Michael R. Lowe et al., "Personal History of Dieting and Family History of Obesity Are Unrelated: Implications for Understanding Weight Gain Proneness," *Eating Behaviors* 17 (2015): doi.org/10.1016/j.eatbeh.2015.01.002.

p. 78   Dieting definitely doesn't work and won't necessarily make you any healthier: Harriet Brown, "The Weight of the Evidence," *Slate*, March 24, 2015, slate.com/technology/2015/03/diets-do-not-work-the-thin-evidence-that-losing-weight-makes-you-healthier.html.

p. 78   No, honestly—diets *really* don't work: Philippe Jacquet et al., "How Dieting Might Make Some Fatter: Modeling Weight Cycling Toward Obesity From a Perspective of Body Composition Autoregulation," *International Journal of Obesity* 44, no. 6 (2020): doi.org/10.1038/s41366-020-0547-1.

p. 78   Body dysmorphic disorder: Kristin Mack and Berit Grøholt, "Dysmorfofobi—nytt lys på gammel sykdom," *Tidsskriftet*, March 20, 2003, tidsskriftet.no/2003/03/oversiktsartikkel/dysmorfofobi-nytt-lys-pa-gammel-sykdom.

p. 79   Ina Luna Gundersen is sent death threats for letting her body hair grow: Sara Boquist, "Ina (25) lot hårene gro—får trusler," *Minmote*, October 27, 2020, minmote.no/nyheter/a/9OoMbl/ina-25-lot-haarene-gro-faar-trusler. Another body-hair positivity activist is American dancer Macey Duff: Jess Hardiman, "Teenage Dancer Embraces Her Body Hair Despite Strangers' Backlash," LAD Bible, February 4, 2020, ladbible.com/news/news-us-teenager-embraces-her-body-hair-despite-strangers-backlash-20200204.

p. 80   Jean Baudrillard: *The Consumer Society: Myths and Structures*, trans. J.P. Mayer (Sage Publications, 1998).

p. 82   More on eating disorders: for muscle dysmorphia in boys, see Kristian Meinich-Bache, "Muskeldysmorfi hos menn med medlemskap på treningssenter—En undersøkelse av utbredelse og potensielle korrelater," University of Agder, thesis, 2019, uia.brage.unit.no/uia-xmlui/bitstream/handle/11250/2620247/Meinich-Bache%2C%20Kristian.pdf?sequence=1&isAllowed=y;

see also Villa Sult (eating disorders institute): spiseforstyrrelser.no/disorders/forekomster-2/; for the rise in eating disorders among boys, see Christina Halvorsen, "Mer spiseforstyrrelser blant men," Dinside, updated September 5, 2016, dinside.no/okonomi/mer-spiseforstyrrelser-blant-menn/62101206.

Step Five: Give the Gorilla a Name

p. 86   Henrik Ibsen: *A Doll's House*, ed. E. Haldeman-Julius (The Floating Press, 2008).

p. 88   The invisible gorilla: Christopher Chabris and Daniel Simons, "Selective Attention Test (1999)," (video), 1:21, The Invisible Gorilla, theinvisiblegorilla.com/gorilla_experiment.html; also mentioned in Hilde Østby and Ylva Østby, *Adventures in Memory: The Science and Secrets of Remembering and Forgetting,* trans. Marianne Lindvall (Greystone, 2018), where we also write about memory in general and depression.

p. 89   Girls and boys learn different things and are asked different questions: Hilde Moi Østbø, "Barnehageansatte behandler jenter og gutter forskjellig," *Stavanger Aftenblad*, October 19, 2017, aftenbladet.no/lokalt/i/Ed4E2/barnehageansatte-behandler-jenter-og-gutter-forskjellig?fbclid=IwAR3HiX1r9TL7aszsKNnbeDJvuvDh nzDudzcerwiHCylxyF5cvgxvqoqMyu4; see "Gender Differences in the Classroom" in "Chapter 4: Student Diversity," Educational Psychology (course), Lumen Learning, courses.lumenlearning.com/suny-educationalpsychology/chapter/gender-differences-in-the-classroom/; for differences in how we teach kids about nature based on their gender, see Helene Uri, *Hvem sa hva? Kvinner, menn og språk* (Gyldendal, 2018).

p. 90   Torkil Færø: *Kamerakuren: Slik du takler øyeblikket, takler du alt* (Cappelen Damm, 2019).

p. 90   Mirror neurons and bibliotherapy, dealt with in Hilde Østby: *The Key to Creativity: The Science Behind Ideas and How Daydreaming Can Change the World*, trans. Matt Bagguley (Greystone, 2023).

p. 92   Depression and anxiety: Johann Hari, *Lost Connections: Why You're Depressed and How to Find Hope* (Bloomsbury, 2019).

p. 93   Sexual abuse and negative body image: Ann Kearney-Cooke and Diann M. Ackard, "The Effects of Sexual Abuse on Body Image, Self-Image, and Sexual Activity of Women," *Journal of Gender-Specific Medicine* 3, no. 6 (2000): pubmed.ncbi.nlm.nih.gov/11253384/; for the link between childhood sexual abuse and

obesity, see Olga Khazan, "The Second Assault," *The Atlantic*,
December 15, 2015, theatlantic.com/health/archive/2015/12/
sexual-abuse-victims-obesity/420186/.

p. 93   Vincent Felitti found that 55 percent of his patients had experienced
sexual abuse during their childhood or youth. That is far higher
than the percentage in the general population. Childhood trauma
is a major cause of morbid obesity; see Jane Ellen Stevens, "Toxic
Stress From Childhood Trauma Causes Obesity, Too," ACES Too
High, May 23, 2012, acestoohigh.com/2012/05/23/toxic-stress-from-
childhood-trauma-causes-obesity-too/. For the original ACE study,
involving almost ten thousand subjects, see Vincent J. Felitti et
al., "Relationship of Childhood Abuse and Household Dysfunction
to Many of the Leading Causes of Death in Adults. The Adverse
Childhood Experiences (ACE) Study," *American Journal of Preventive
Medicine* 14, no. 4 (1998), doi.org/10.1016/s0749-3797(98)00017-8.

p. 94   The risk factors that increase the likelihood of addiction by
4600 percent: Johann Hari, "Childhood Trauma & Addiction: The
4600% Risk Factor," openDemocracy, July 19, 2015, opendemocracy
.net/en/childhood-trauma-addiction-4600-risk-factor/.

p. 94   On body image and rape: Inbar Kremer et al., "Body Image Among
Victims of Sexual and Physical Abuse," *Violence and Victims* 28, no. 2
(2013): doi.org/10.1891/0886-6708.vv-D-12-00015.

p. 94   In this study, eight hundred of the sixteen hundred participants
had experienced rape: Ann Kearney-Cooke and Diann M. Ackard,
"The Effects of Sexual Abuse on Body Image, Self-Image, and Sexual
Activity of Women," *Journal of Gender-Specific Medicine* 3, no. 6
(2000): pubmed.ncbi.nlm.nih.gov/11253384/.

p. 94   The Norwegian police's rape report: *Voldtektssituasjonen 2019*,
Kripos, October 2020, politiet.no/globalassets/04-aktuelt-tall-
og-fakta/voldtekt-og-seksuallovbrudd/voldtektssituasjonen-i-
norge-2019.pdf.

p. 94   The Norwegian Centre for Violence and Traumatic Stress Studies
(NKVTS) reported in 2023 that 22 percent of all Norwegian women
have been raped one or more times in the course of their lives,
half of them before they turned eighteen: See "Høy forekomst av
vold og overgrep i Norge," Nasjonalt kunnskapssenter om vold
og traumatisk stress, February 28, 2023, nkvts.no/aktuelt/hoy-
forekomst-av-vold-og-overgrep-i-norge/. In terms of US statistics,
according to the organization RAINN (Rape, Abuse & Incest
National Network), "1 out of every 6 American women has been the
victim of an attempted or completed rape in her lifetime

(14.8% completed, 2.8% attempted)." See "Scope of the Problem: Statistics," RAINN, rainn.org/statistics/scope-problem.

p. 95   Benedict de Spinoza: *Ethics* (Hafner Publishing Company, 1949).

Step Six: Stress Less

p. 99   The sympathetic and parasympathetic nervous systems: Siw Aduvill, *Hvil: Alt vi vinner ved å la være* (Tiden, 2019).

p. 100   Stress and the primitive brain: Amy Arnsten et al., "Everyday Stress Can Shut Down the Brain's Chief Command Center," *Scientific American* 306, no. 4 (2012): doi.org/10.1038/scientificamerican0412-48.

p. 100   More on stress: Anne Gunn Halvorsen, *Stress og korleis leve med det* (Samlaget, 2019).

p. 100   Stress and corticotropin-releasing hormone: Sally Robertson, "Obesity and Stress," News Medical, updated December 22, 2022, news-medical.net/health/Obesity-and-stress.aspx.

p. 101   The brain's "daydreaming mode": Hilde Østby, *The Key to Creativity: The Science Behind Ideas and How Daydreaming Can Change the World*, trans. Matt Bagguley (Greystone, 2023).

p. 103   Cornaro's diet book: Conor Heffernan, "Diet Advice From the 16th Century," Physical Culture Study, November 12, 2015, physicalculturestudy.com/2015/11/12/diet-advice-from-the-16th-century.

p. 104   On deep breathing: Audun Myskja, *Pust: Nøkkelen til styrke, helse og glede* (Stenersens Forlag, 2018).

p. 104   On the vagus nerve, and breathing and smiling: Siw Aduvill, *Hvil: Alt vi vinner ved å la være* (Tiden, 2019).

p. 105   Laughter yoga: Laughter Yoga International, laughteryoga.org/.

p. 107   On Prozac's history: Anna Moore, "Eternal Sunshine," *The Guardian*, May 13, 2007, theguardian.com/society/2007/may/13/socialcare.medicineandhealth.

p. 108   Rising use of antidepressants: Lea Winerman, "By the Numbers: Antidepressant Use on the Rise," *Monitor on Psychology* 48, no. 10 (2017): apa.org/monitor/2017/11/numbers; for Prozac use in the United States, see "Fluoxetine," ClinCalc.com, clincalc.com/DrugStats/Drugs/Fluoxetine.

p. 108   Growth in antidepressant use among young people: "Percentage of Teenagers in the United States Taking Antidepressants From

2015 to 2019, by Gender," Statista, April 2020, statista.com/
statistics/1133612/antidepressant-use-teenagers-by-gender-
us/#:~:text=Antidepressant%20use%20among%20teenagers%20
in,from%202015%2D2019%2C%20by%20gender&text=Based%2-
0on%20pharmacy%20claims%20of,antidepressants%20compared%20
to%20teenage%20boys; Matt Richtel, "'It's Life or Death': The Mental
Health Crisis Among U.S. Teens," *New York Times*, April 24, 2022,
nytimes.com/2022/04/23/health/mental-health-crisis-teens.html.

p. 108   Joanna Moncrieff on antidepressants: Knut-Øyvind Hagen and
          David Vojislav Krekling, "Antidepressiva virker ikke, og gir en
          generasjon av hjelpeløs ungdom," NRK, updated November 16, 2018,
          nrk.no/norge/_-antidepressiva-virker-ikke_-og-gir-en-generasjon-
          av-hjelpelos-ungdom-1.14292443.

p. 108   Antidepressants—why they don't work and what actually does:
          Johann Hari, *Lost Connections: Why You're Depressed and How to
          Find Hope* (Bloomsbury, 2019).

p. 109   Cortisol levels in hair and morbid obesity: Mary Caffrey,
          "Measuring Cortisol Levels in Hair Shows Link Between Stress,
          Obesity," *American Journal of Managed Care*, February 27, 2017,
          ajmc.com/view/measuring-cortisol-levels-in-hair-shows-link-
          between-stress-obesity.

p. 110   Stress hormones and our sedentary lifestyle: Siw Aduvill, *Hvile: Alt
          vi vinner ved å la være* (Tiden, 2019).

p. 110   Obesity: Hannah Ritchie and Max Roser, "Obesity," Our World in
          Data, 2017, ourworldindata.org/obesity; John Komlos and Marek
          Brabec, "The Evolution of BMI Values of US Adults: 1882–1986,"
          VoxEU, Centre for Economic Policy Research, August 31, 2010,
          voxeu.org/article/100-years-us-obesity.

p. 111   Facts about depression: Martin Steen Tesli, "Psykiske plager og
          lidelser hos voksne," Folkehelseinstituttet, updated April 17, 2023,
          fhi.no/nettpub/hin/psykisk-helse/psykiske-lidelser-voksne/;
          "Depressive Disorder (Depression)," World Health Organization,
          March 31, 2023, who.int/news-room/fact-sheets/detail/
          depression; Saloni Dattani, "What Is the Lifetime Risk of
          Depression?" Our World in Data, May 18, 2022, ourworldindata
          .org/depression-lifetime-risk.

p. 113   Humanity's evolution: Erin Wayman, "Rethinking Modern Human
          Origins," *Smithsonian Magazine*, July 23, 2012, smithsonianmag
          .com/science-nature/rethinking-modern-human-origins-5370343/.

p. 114   Haredi Jews: as discussed in Noreena Hertz, *The Lonely Century:
          Coming Together in a World That's Pulling Apart* (Sceptre, 2020).

p. 114   Maria Borelius writes about "the blue zones": *Health Revolution: Finding Happiness and Health Through an Anti-Inflammatory Lifestyle*, trans. Sonia Wichmann (Harper Design, 2019); and in *Bliss: De nye antiinflammatoriske nøklene til et lengre og bedre liv*, trans. Lisbeth Kristoffersen (Pilar, 2020).

p. 114   Rats and stroking: Susannah C. Walker et al., "C-Low Threshold Mechanoafferent Targeted Dynamic Touch Modulates Stress Resilience in Rats Exposed to Chronic Mild Stress," *European Journal of Neuroscience* 55, nos. 9–10 (2022): doi.org/10.1111/ejn.14951.

p. 114   C-tactile afferents: Ralph Pawling et al., "C-Tactile Afferent Stimulating Touch Carries a Positive Affective Value," *PLOS One* 12, no. 3 (2017): doi.org/10.1371/journal.pone.0173457.

p. 116   Daydreaming, memory, visions of the future, and depression, as well as research on reading and mirror neurons, and all the research on forest hikes: Hilde Østby, *The Key to Creativity: The Science Behind Ideas and How Daydreaming Can Change the World*, trans. Matt Bagguley (Greystone, 2023).

p. 118   The average eight-year-old and their relationship to nature: Anne Sverdrup-Thygeson, *Tapestries of Life: Uncovering the Lifesaving Secrets of the Natural World*, trans. Lucy Moffatt (Mudlark, 2020).

p. 118   Neurologist Oliver Sacks on gardens as medicine and inspiration: "Oliver Sacks: The Healing Power of Gardens," *New York Times*, April 18, 2019, nytimes.com/2019/04/18/opinion/sunday/oliver-sacks-gardens.html.

p. 119   Research shows that people who live or spend time close to nature are less prone to depression: Johann Hari, *Lost Connections: Why You're Depressed and How to Find Hope* (Bloomsbury, 2019).

p. 119   Sam Everington and gardens: "Nourishing the Nation's Soul Since 1927," Investec, October 5, 2020, investec.com/en_gb/focus/at-home/Gardens-and-health.html.

p. 119   Johann Hari on gardening as an antidepressant: Johann Hari, "We Need New Ways of Treating Depression," *Vox*, updated June 13, 2018, vox.com/the-big-idea/2018/2/25/16997572/causes-depression-pills-prozac-social-environmental-connections-hari. More on gardening to treat anxiety and depression can be found in Peter A. Coventry et al., "Nature-Based Outdoor Activities for Mental and Physical Health: Systematic Review and Meta-Analysis," *SSM—Population Health* 16 (2021): doi.org/10.1016/j.ssmph.2021.100934 and "Gardening May Help Reduce Cancer Risk and Boost Mental Health," *Neuroscience News*, January 6, 2023, neurosciencenews.com/gardening-mental-health-cancer-22190/.

p. 119 On bacteria and the brain: Erik Martiniussen, *Krigen mot bakteriene: Helsekrisen som truer oss og hvordan vi kan løse den* (Press, 2020); Juliet Landrø, "Bakterier styrer hjernen," Forskning.no, February 8, 2011, forskning.no/hjernen/bakterier-styrer-hjernen/795036; Gorm Palmgren, "Bakterier i hjernen gjør deg glad," Illustrert Vitenskap, September 12, 2022, illvit.no/mennesket/hjernen-medisin/bakterier-i-hjernen-gjoer-deg-glad.

p. 120 The sea and the BlueHealth research project: Elle Hunt, "Blue Spaces: Why Time Spent Near Water Is the Secret of Happiness," *The Guardian*, November 3, 2019, theguardian.com/lifeandstyle/2019/nov/03/blue-space-living-near-water-good-secret-of-happiness. See also the project's website at bluehealth2020.eu/.

p. 121 On telomeres, inflammations, sunsets, and "awe": Maria Borelius, *Health Revolution: Finding Happiness and Health Through an Anti-Inflammatory Lifestyle*, trans. Sonia Wichmann (Harper Design, 2019); and *Bliss: De nye antiinflammatoriske nøklene til et lengre og bedre liv*, trans. Lisbeth Kristoffersen (Pilar, 2020).

Step Seven: I Become Free, One Breath at a Time

p. 125 William Shakespeare: *Romeo and Juliet* (Penguin Books, 2016).

p. 126 Research into eye contact: Hilde Østby, *The Key to Creativity: The Science Behind Ideas and How Daydreaming Can Change the World*, trans. Matt Bagguley (Greystone, 2023).

p. 127 On Henry Solomon Wellcome: "Henry Wellcome," Wikipedia, en.wikipedia.org/wiki/Henry_Wellcome; John Launer, "Henry Wellcome: The Man Who Made Medicine," *Postgraduate Medical Journal* 93, no. 1102 (2017): doi.org/10.1136/postgradmedj-2017-135182.

p. 130 Hermit beetles: Anne Sverdrup-Thygeson, *Tapestries of Life: Uncovering the Lifesaving Secrets of the Natural World*, trans. Lucy Moffatt (Mudlark, 2020).

p. 131 On the elements contained in our bodies: read more in Anja Røyne, *The Elements We Live By: How Iron Helps Us Breathe, Potassium Lets Us See, and Other Surprising Superpowers of the Periodic Table*, trans. Olivia Lasky (The Experiment, 2020).

p. 132 Derek Walcott's poem "Love After Love": originally published in the collection *Sea Grapes* (FSG, 1976).

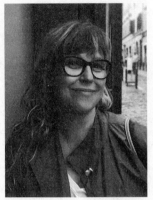

MATT BAGGULEY

About the Author

HILDE ØSTBY is an author, journalist, and a historian of ideas. After debuting in 2013 with the critically acclaimed novel *Encyclopedia of Longing*, she went on to write the international nonfiction bestseller *Adventures in Memory* with her sister Ylva, followed by *The Key to Creativity*. Her books have been translated into twenty different languages. She lives in Oslo, Norway.